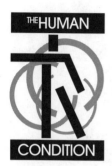

The Human Condition

Study Guide

Fourth Edition

by

Wendy Schiff

prepared by

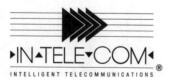

INTELLIGENT TELECOMMUNICATIONS

JONES AND BARTLETT PUBLISHERS

Sudbury, Massachusetts

BOSTON   TORONTO   LONDON   SINGAPORE

The Human Condition is a television- and web-based course produced by INTELECOM Intelligent Telecommunications

Essential Concepts for Healthy Living, Fourth Edition, by Jones and Bartlett Publishers is the text designated for use with this course, in conjunction with the video programs and this study guide.

Printed in the United States of America
09 08 07 06 05   10 9 8 7 6 5 4 3 2 1

ISBN 0-7637-3725-9

For more information contact Jones and Bartlett Publishers, 40 Tall Pine Drive, Sudbury, MA 01776 or visit our web site at www.jbpub.com.

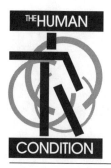

Contents

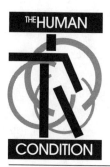

Introduction

The Human Condition is a fascinating and compelling telecourse that explores the major health concerns and issues that we face at the beginning of the twenty-first century. Scientific research, technological advancements, and a systematic approach to medical education make the health care system in the United States among the best in the world. Nevertheless, heart disease, cancer, obesity, hypertension, and diabetes affect the lives of most Americans. These serious conditions are largely the result of lifestyle choices. A major goal of the developers of *The Human Condition* and the authors of the textbook *Essential Concepts for Healthy Living* is to make you more aware of the various factors, including lifestyle, that affect health.

The Human Condition introduces you to a number of health care professionals who are experts in their fields. These individuals were willing to make time in their busy schedules to participate in the production of this teleweb-course. They graciously welcomed INTELECOM staff, including writers, directors, researchers, and camera crews, into their workplaces. You also will meet people who are living "The Human Condition." These individuals have made or are making major decisions that concern their health and well-being. They were willing to discuss their experiences with you, in the hopes that you will learn more about health and health care from them.

The Course

The Human Condition course presents the latest information about health, including information about medical technologies and innovative treatments that affect you now or are likely to affect you in the future. In addition to your on-campus instructor, *The Human Condition* course includes three complementary educational elements: 26 half-hour videos; this study guide; and the new and revised fourth edition of the popular and critically-acclaimed textbook, *Essential Concepts for Healthy Living*, by Sandra Alters and Wendy Schiff. This textbook has been chosen to accompany the course because it is well-researched, well-written, and up-to-date. Included with the textbook is a student workbook that contains decision making and assessment activities.

To find more helpful learning activities that accompany the textbook, visit the publisher's website (http://www.jbpub.com/healthyliving). This site includes the following resources and learning tools:

○ **Practice Quizzes** comprised of 15 multiple choice questions derived from the Instructor's Manual that accompanies *Essential Concepts for Healthy Living.*

○ **Animated Flashcards** for defining terms used in each chapter of the textbook.

○ **Healthy People 2010 Updates** that provide information concerning Americans' progress toward meeting national health goals.

○ **Content Links** for Web sites that provide additional resources for reliable health information.

○ **Web Exercises** provide additional sources on the Internet for the information covered in the text and related study opportunities.

○ An **Interactive Glossary** provides the ability to look up the definitions of terms used in the text by searching for the word or by browsing terms alphabetically or by text chapter.

The Study Guide

Learning about health is a challenging yet rewarding task. The amount of health information that covers the numerous broad but interrelated topics sometimes can seem unmanageable. This study guide is designed to help you prepare to watch *The Human Condition* and study for examinations that cover information in course.

This guide includes a lesson for each of the half-hour video shows. Each lesson has the following features:

○ **Learning Objectives** that identify what you should be able to do after viewing the videotape and reading the required selections from the textbook. Many test bank questions are derived from these objectives.

○ An **Overview** that summarizes the lesson's main topics.

○ **Assignments** that link the video lesson with related sections of the textbook.

○ **Key Terms** and their definitions that help you learn the "language" of health.

○ **Video Viewing Questions** that help you follow and analyze information in the video and integrate the information with your readings.

○ **Expanded Analysis** activities or questions that help you think critically about the information presented in the video.

○ A **Self-Test** that enables you to check your understanding of the material in the videos and textbook. The format of self-test questions is similar to questions in the instructor's test bank.

Self-Test Questions

Every lesson includes a set of questions covering material in the video and assigned textbook readings. Each self-test has multiple choice and short answer questions; some self-tests include matching questions. An answer key is provided, and if the answer is in the textbook, page numbers are shown to indicate where you can find it.

Before you view the video lessons, follow the "Assignments" listed in the guide. As you read the textbook, highlight key information and review *Healthy Living Practices*, chapter summaries, and key terms. The chapters include at least one of the following boxes: *Managing Your Health, Consumer Health,* and *Diversity in Health.* Be sure to read the boxed materials; these features contain interesting and useful information, and test questions may cover this material.

It is a good idea to watch each episode completely and without taking notes. Then view the episode a second time, taking notes as you watch. If you would like to refer to episodes at a later date, you may videotape them for your use only.

After viewing each episode, take some time to review your notes while the information is still fresh in your mind. Do not wait until the day before an exam to review your notes. If you do not understand a concept, use the index to locate where the concept is discussed in the textbook. If you still have questions concerning this material, write them down in the guide and contact your instructor.

You are encouraged to check your answers against the answer keys after you take each classroom exam or quiz. Review information in the textbook or your notes that is related to the items you missed. Then, if you still have questions or would like additional information, be sure to check with your instructor. The tests can be a valuable part of your learning if you take the time to review your performance and strengthen any weak areas.

Video Episodes

1. The Fabric of Health
2. In Human Terms
3. State of Mind
4. Lives in Balance
5. Behind Closed Doors
6. It's Personal
7. Risky Business
8. The Code
9. Haley or Matthew's Story
10. The Growing Years
11. Web of Addiction
12. Feels so Good (Hurts so Bad)
13. What You Don't Know...
14. Food for Thought
15. Weighing In
16. Working it Out
17. Germ Warfare
18. The Modern Plague
19. Heart of the Matter
20. Brain Attack
21. Diagnosis Cancer
22. Living with Cancer
23. Age Happens
24. Final Chapter
25. The Medical Marketplace
26. What Price?

Summary of Reading Assignments

in *Essential Concepts for Healthy Living*, 4th edition, by Alters and Schiff

Study Guide Lesson	Text Assignment
1. The Fabric of Health	— Chapter 1, "Health: The Foundation for Life"
2. In Human Terms	— No reading assignment in the text
3. State of Mind	— Chapter 2, "Psychological Health"
4. Lives in Balance	— Chapter 3, "Stress and Its Management" — Review the section on post traumatic stress disorder in Chapter 2, page 38
5. Behind Closed Doors	— Chapter 4, "Violence and Abuse"
6. It's Personal	— Chapter 6, "Relationships and Sexuality"
7. Risky Business	— Chapter 5, "Reproductive Health" — Chapter 14, "Infection, Immunity, and Noninfectious Disease," pages 398–415 — Review Chapter 6, pages 136–139
8. The Code	— Chapter 14, "Infection, Immunity, and Noninfectious Disease," pages 379–379 and review 413–415
9. Haley or Matthew's Story	— Review Chapter 5, "Reproductive Health," pages 102–112 — Chapter 9, "Across the Lifespan" section, pages 248–251
10. The Growing Years	— No reading assignment in the text
11. Web of Addiction	— Chapter 7, "Drug Use and Abuse"
12. Feels so Good (Hurts so Bad)	— Chapter 8, "Alcohol and Tobacco"
13. What You Don't Know…	— Chapter 16, "Environmental Health"
14. Food for Thought	— Chapter 9, "Nutrition"
15. Weighing In	— Chapter 10, "Body Weight and Its Management"
16. Working it Out	— Chapter 11, "Physical Fitness"
17. Germ Warfare	— Chapter 14, "Infection, Immunity, and Noninfectious Disease"
18. The Modern Plague	— Review Chapter 14, pages 398–403
19. Heart of the Matter	— Chapter 12, "Cardiovascular Health"
20. Brain Attack	— Review Chapter 12, "Cardiovascular Health"
21. Diagnosis Cancer	— Chapter 13, "Cancer"
22. Living with Cancer	— Review Chapter 13
23. Age Happens	— Chapter 15, "Aging, Dying, and Death," especially pages 423–433
24. Final Chapter	— Review Chapter 15, especially pages 433–447
25. The Medical Marketplace	— No reading assignment in the text
26. What Price?	— No reading assignment in the text

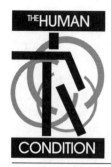

1

The Fabric of Health

Learning Objectives

Upon completing this lesson, you should be familiar with the facts and concepts presented in the lesson and should be able to:

○ Explain why the definitions of health encompass more than just physical health.

○ Discuss how heredity and environment interact to influence a person's health and life expectancy.

○ Give examples of statistical measures used to determine the health status of a group of people or nation.

○ Compare U. S. health statistics to those of other industrialized nations and suggest reasons for the differences that exist.

○ Recognize the effects that lifestyle choices can have on health and life expectancy.

○ Evaluate at least three sources of information on a health topic of interest to you.

Overview

Physical health is only one aspect of health. Most experts view health as a positive state that encompasses multiple aspects of the individual, including physical, psychological, and social dimensions. These dimensions interact with each other, influencing each person's health and well-being. As a result, a healthy individual is a productive member of society.

Genetic, social, political, and environmental factors play important roles in determining the quality of one's health. But economic factors influence who has access to the best medical care, gets immunizations, has nutritious food, and drinks clean water. In the United States, for example, the population expects local, state, and federal governments to provide a variety of health-related services, such as monitoring water quality and regulating food safety and drug purity. The government also provides a variety of public health programs for Americans, especially those with low incomes. Such programs emphasize the importance of preventive healthcare, including prenatal care, infant checkups, and immunizations. Although Americans generally have long life expectancies, the rising cost of healthcare is a major barrier to those who need that care the most: children and the elderly.

What affects the health and well-being of people in poor countries will eventually affect the health and well-being of people in wealthy countries. Donald Hopkins, physician and Associate Executive Director of the Carter Center, says, "...[the world] is one small boat...it's in our interest to help everybody understand their health and deal with their health problems...." Thus, health is a global concern, and we are all in the "same boat."

Statistical Evidence for Health

The life expectancy of a population reflects the number of people who die early in life. Compared to other developed countries, infant mortality is high in the United States. When a relatively high number of infants die in a population, the life expectancy for the entire population drops. But why is the infant mortality rate high in the United States? Lack of health insurance is a major barrier to any American who needs medical care; low-income women often lack adequate health insurance to pay for prenatal visits. However, using infant mortality as a measure of the quality of health care in a country may provide misleading information about the state of the nation's healthcare system. According to Dr. William Schwartz, Professor of Medicine, University of Southern California, "...it's quite unfair to judge a system on the basis solely of length of life and infant mortality." Dr. Schwartz points out that much of what modern medical technology has been able to achieve has improved the quality of our lives without appreciably extending our life expectancies. Although "quality of life" is a positive outcome, it is difficult to measure objectively.

A Matter of Responsibility

Everyone needs to take personal responsibility for their own health. Improving one's health and lengthening one's life expectancy may be as simple as changing a single behavior, such as stopping smoking. Dr. Hopkins says, "The key understanding is that what I do affects my health at least as much, maybe more, than anything that can be done to me in a hospital... I need to...start taking care of my health right from a very young age...[Young people need to understand that] some of the decisions they're making...affect them for the rest of their lives."

Assignments

○ Read Chapter 1, "Health: The Foundation for Life," in Alters & Schiff, *Essential Concepts for Healthy Living*, 4th edition. You may find it helpful to take notes on your reading. Then read the Learning Objectives and Overview for this lesson. Review the Key Terms below.

○ Scan the Video Viewing Questions, and then watch the video program for Lesson 1, "The Fabric of Health."

○ After watching the video, answer the Video Viewing Questions and assess your learning with the Self-Test.

○ Complete the activities for Chapter 1 in the workbook that accompanies the textbook. Your instructor may use these activities as assignments.

Key Terms

The following terms and those defined in Chapter 1 are important to your understanding of this unit.

angioplasty	— The reconstruction of damaged blood vessels.
HMO	— Acronym for health maintenance organizations, providers of healthcare in the United States.
infrastructure	— Basic facilities and services needed for the growth, functioning, and maintenance of a country.
morbidity	— The incidence of disease in a population.
PAHO	— Acronym for Pan-American Health Organization, an international organization that promotes health efforts for people living in the Americas.
oral rehydration therapy	— Treatment for dehydration that involves drinking watery fluids.

Video Viewing Questions

1. The term "health" is difficult to define. The experts in "The Fabric of Health" provide their own definitions of health. What elements of health do they mention? What role do a person's genes play in influencing his or her health?

2. In the United States, poor people do not enjoy the same quality of life and health as people with high incomes. How does a country's "economic well-being" affect the health of its people? What is the U.S. government doing to safeguard the health of Americans?

3. In general, people with low incomes are not concerned with preventive health care needs, such as having routine health checkups and making sure their children are immunized. Why is preventive care not a priority of people with low incomes?

4. What is a major emphasis of the World Health Organization and its related organization, the Pan-American Health Organization? What are some of the leading causes of death in developing countries? In the future, what conditions are likely to be among the leading causes of death in these nations?

5. Many Americans face barriers when they need health care. What are some of these barriers? Which industrialized nations have large numbers of people who do not have health insurance?

6. Americans cannot rely on their government to take care of every health problem, especially conditions that are the result of unhealthy lifestyles. What can each American do to take responsibility for his or her health?

Self-Test

Multiple Choice

1. According to health experts Peter Clarke and David Bennet, which of the following statements is the best definition of "health"?
   a. Health is having a body that is not diseased, weak, or defective.
   b. Health is not being sick or weak, having friends, and feeling good about yourself.
   c. Health is having the ability to be productive, creative, and active while enjoying life.
   d. Health is having the physical strength and emotional commitment to live a long life.

2. Which of the following groups of Americans has the highest risk of poor health?
   a. College students
   b. The poor
   c. People who have Asian ancestry
   d. Health care practitioners

3. What is a major cause of illness in the United States?
   a. Poor air quality.
   b. Pesticide residues on food.
   c. Inadequately sanitized water.
   d. Smoking cigarettes.

4. According to Dr. Clarke, people with limited incomes sacrifice _____ first, so they'll have enough money to meet their basic needs.
   a. nutritious food
   b. rental housing payments
   c. car payments
   d. vacations

5. Economic conditions influence one's access to quality health care. In the United States, which segments of the low-income population are most likely to suffer because of limited access to health care?
   a. Middle-aged women
   b. College students
   c. Elderly people
   d. Middle-aged men

6. Which of the following organizations provides an international forum for sharing information about infectious diseases and coordinates efforts to control or eradicate them?
   a. The International Agency on Human Health
   b. The Multinational Health Federation
   c. The Health Consortium of Developing Countries
   d. The World Health Organization

7. In the past, infectious diseases killed or disabled many young Americans. Vaccines for many serious childhood infections are now available, and immunization programs have reduced the prevalence of these diseases in the United States. Under-developed countries, however, have large numbers of people who have not been immunized with these vaccines. Which of the following conditions is an infectious disease that is no longer a problem in the United States because of an effective vaccine, but is still widespread in India and in parts of the Middle East and Africa?
    a. Polio
    b. Cystic fibrosis
    c. Endometriosis
    d. AIDS

8. Ted's great-grandfather was born in 1900. At that time, what was the leading cause of death in the United States?
    a. Suicide
    b. Horseback riding injury
    c. Lung cancer
    d. Tuberculosis

9. Within the next few decades, which of the following behaviors will be the leading cause of death in the world?
    a. Smoking cigarettes
    b. Drinking alcohol
    c. Eating fatty meats
    d. Refusing to wear seat belts

10. In developing countries, infectious diseases are major causes of death. Which of the following infectious diseases is not a major cause of death in these nations?
    a. Measles
    b. Gonorrhea
    c. Malaria
    d. Tuberculosis

11. Dean Hamer, Ph.D. and Chief of Gene Structure and Regulation at the National Cancer Institute, states that our genes determine our physical health and, to some extent, the functioning of our brain. Explain how your genes influence your health.

Short Answer

12. Explain the difference between life span and life expectancy. What factors influence life expectancy?

Expanded Analysis

1. According to Dr. James Curran, the medical community needs a commitment to "primacy and prevention rather than cure." What does he mean?

2. What can local health organizations, hospitals, and health departments do to educate the people in your community about the importance of preventive health care?

3. As tobacco use declines in the United States, cigarette manufacturers have turned to new, less-regulated markets in developing countries. Why do you think the governments of these countries do not seem to be concerned about the long-term risks of tobacco use?

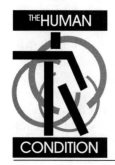

THE HUMAN
CONDITION

2

In Human Terms

Learning Objectives

Upon completing this lesson, you should be familiar with the facts and concepts presented in this lesson and should be able to:

○ Compare the health challenges facing people who live in third-world countries to those you face in everyday life.

○ Address questions regarding why it is important to help support the health status of people who live in distant lands.

○ Recognize how custom and culture impact the role of the medical practitioner and the health of families.

○ Describe the impact that poverty has on access to healthcare services in the United States.

○ List at least three services provided by the Venice Family Clinic that are of particular value to the populations it serves.

Overview

Whether a country is torn apart by civil war and ravaged by famine and disease or is one of the richest, most productive nations in the world, some of its people will suffer from a lack of adequate economic resources. Doctors Without Borders is an organization comprised of physicians from 45 nations who provide medical care to desperate people wherever the need arises. In 1996–1997, for example, Doctors Without Borders provided nutritional support and infectious disease control for starving Somali refugees entering Kenya in Africa. The refugees were suffering from severe malnutrition, which had a particularly devastating impact on the children. In developed countries, children suffering from diarrhea and pneumonia can survive if they receive proper treatment, but in poor, developing countries like Kenya, these infections kill malnourished children.

Healthcare practitioners who are trained in modern methods of treating diseases often face numerous challenges when they try to help sick people in developing nations. Cultural traditions, for example, may interfere with a treatment plan or even spread diseases. Furthermore, the lack of adequate medical supplies and facilities reduces the healthcare practitioner's ability to provide life-saving care.

Although the situation in Venice, California, is vastly different than that of the Somali refugees in Kenya, a growing number of low-income people living in that area lack the resources to obtain adequate medical care. As a result, they depend on the Venice Family Clinic for their basic primary care needs. Many of the patients who use the clinic are recent immigrants or homeless. Typically, they are very sick because they don't take care of themselves, and they haven't had routine medical care because they lack medical insurance.

In the United States, the need for universal medical insurance has been a hotly debated issue for several years. It seems unconscionable that so many uninsured or inadequately insured Americans live in such a wealthy and productive nation. Is this country likely to embrace socialized medicine in the future? Only time will tell.

Assignments

○ Read the Learning Objectives and Overview for this lesson. Review the Key Terms below.

○ Scan the Video Viewing Questions, and then watch the video program for Lesson 2, "In Human Terms."

○ After watching the video, answer the Video Viewing Questions and assess your learning with the Self-Test.

Key Terms

The following terms are important to your understanding of this unit.

asymptomatic	— Having no signs or symptoms of illness.
capitated	— Referring to the practice in managed care programs of reimbursing physicians a set amount for each patient, regardless of the extent of the patient's care.
electrolyte	— An element or compound that can conduct electric current under certain conditions.
nephrology	— The study of the kidney and the conditions that affect it.

Video Viewing Questions

1. What are some challenges that medical practitioners often face when they work in developing countries?

2. What are the physical and behavioral signs of a child who is suffering from starvation? What do these children die from?

3. What is the mission of the Venice Family Clinic? Who does the clinic primarily serve?

4. In many instances, patients are very sick when they come to the Venice Family Clinic. Why don't these patients seek medical care before their illnesses become so serious?

5. How does the quality of medical care at the Venice Family Clinic compare to the care that one receives as a patient who has health insurance and is being treated by a physician in private practice?

Self-Test

1. An international organization committed to serving all populations in need of medical care, regardless of political differences or national boundaries is
   a. the National Health Federation.
   b. Medical Help for Humanity.
   c. Doctors Without Borders.
   d. the International Medical Association.

Multiple Choice

2. The largest free clinic in the United States is
   a. the Venice Family Clinic.
   b. the Monroe County Preventive Healthcare Clinic.
   c. the Chicago Hope Clinic.
   d. the Appalachian Trail Clinic.

3. During the civil war in Somalia, starving children were more likely to die from _____ than other causes.
   a. chickenpox
   b. mumps
   c. influenza
   d. pneumonia

4. Which of the following behaviors is often observed in a child suffering from severe starvation?
   a. Increased appetite
   b. Mental depression
   c. Excessive talking
   d. Walking aimlessly in circles

5. Why does cholera kill so rapidly?
   a. Cholera weakens the person's immune system so they develop numerous deadly infections.
   b. Cholera reduces the blood supply to the lungs so the person stops breathing.
   c. Cholera causes severe loss of body water as a result of diarrhea and vomiting.
   d. Cholera increases blood pressure to such high levels that arteries rupture.

6. What is the mission of the Venice Family Clinic?

   a. Provide comprehensive primary health care that's affordable for low-income people who have no health insurance.

   b. Provide 24-hour a day, emergency care to everyone who has health insurance.

   c. Provide tertiary medical care, including in-patient drug rehabilitation programs, for low-income, working class people.

   d. Provide affordable hospital care, including in-patient surgeries and intensive care for seriously ill newborns, children, and adults.

7. According to Susan Fleischman, medical director of the Venice Family Clinic, the people who use the Clinic are "very, very sick." Which of the following conditions are commonly diagnosed or treated in people who use the Clinic's medical services?

   a. Hypertension

   b. Hypervitaminosis

   c. Eclampsia

   d. Cystic fibrosis

Short Answer

8. Physicians who participate in "Doctors Without Borders" face many obstacles to providing adequate care for their patients. Discuss at least three of those obstacles.

9. Healthcare practitioners who work at the Venice Family Clinic also face many obstacles to providing adequate care for their patients. Discuss two of those obstacles.

10. Explain why so many of the patients treated at the Venice Family Clinic are very sick when they come in for care.

Expanded Analysis

1. Several Somali children who were being treated at the Doctors Without Borders clinic died when a cholera epidemic spread through the facility. The parents wanted to bury their dead children according to Islamic religious practices. Why were the physicians concerned about returning the bodies to their parents?

2. Traditional health care practices often conflict with Western medical practices. As recent immigrants from cultures that rely on traditional healing methods adjust to living in the United States, what problems do their cultural backgrounds pose for Western medical practitioners?

3. What are the problems associated with universal health care coverage? Why do some Americans oppose government efforts to socialize medical care in the United States?

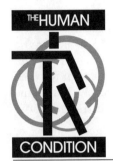

THE HUMAN CONDITION

3

State of Mind

Learning Objectives

Upon completing this lesson, you should be familiar with the facts and concepts presented in the lesson and should be able to:

○ Describe the characteristics of a psychologically healthy person.

○ Compare the prevalence, cost, and understanding of mental health disorders to other major types of illness.

○ Explore factors that contribute to the development of psychological disorders.

○ Identify common mental health disorders, their symptoms, and treatment.

○ Discuss causal factors related to the eating disorders bulimia and anorexia nervosa, and treatments that have proven effective.

Overview

Psychologically healthy people accept themselves, enjoy life, and have the skills to engage the world in ways that are meaningful. One in five Americans, however, has some form of mental illness. Having a mental illness such as depression or schizophrenia interferes with one's ability to be sociable and productive and to enjoy life.

The factors that cause mental illnesses are complex. Some disorders are the result of a disease or injury that damages the brain. In many instances, the abnormal behavior occurs when one responds to difficult life situations. Additionally, abnormal or problematic behavior can be the result of one's personality or family history.

Treatment for mental illness may include individual and group counseling, psychotherapy, and medication. For some people with psychological problems, counseling helps them understand their condition and find solutions to their problems. Others benefit from a combination of medication and therapy. Table 2-5 in the textbook lists the types of mental health specialists who may provide counseling or psychotherapy and describes the training they receive; Table 2-6 lists medications that are frequently prescribed in the treatment of psychological disorders.

Although physicians have effective therapies that often can improve the quality of life for people with mental illness, many people choose not to use them. Dr. Andrew Leuchter, at the Neuropsychiatric Institute and Hospital, University of California–Los Angeles, notes, "...patients don't want to come in for treatment. They feel they're being labeled." Unfortunately, the stigma attached to being labeled "mentally ill" can act as a major barrier for those who might benefit from treatment.

Eating Disorders

Although many people think eating disorders are nutritional problems, individuals who suffer from these disabling conditions have underlying psychological disturbances, especially mood and anxiety disorders. Dr. Michael Strober, Director of the Eating Disorders Program at the University of California–Los Angeles, notes, "...the feared object—that which is phobically avoided—is body shape, body fat. It's a morbid dread of body fat." The obvious difference between a person with anorexia nervosa and one with bulimia nervosa is body shape. The person with anorexia nervosa starves herself and looks emaciated. The person with bulimia nervosa overeats but maintains normal body weight, usually by vomiting after overeating. Both illnesses are treated with medication, psychotherapy, and nutritional counseling.

Today's approaches to treatment often can help people affected by psychological disorders to lead normal lives. Unfortunately, many individuals do not seek treatment because they cannot overcome the stigma of mental illness. As more people with these conditions come forward and describe their positive responses to treatment, perhaps more people will be willing to seek the help they so desperately need.

Assignments

○ Read Chapter 2, "Psychological Health," in Alters & Schiff, *Essential Concepts for Healthy Living*, 4th edition. You may find it helpful to take notes on your reading. Then read the Learning Objectives and Overview for this lesson. Review the Key Terms below.

○ Scan the Video Viewing Questions, and then watch the video program for Lesson 3, "State of Mind."

○ After watching the video, answer the Video Viewing Questions and assess your learning with the Self-Test.

○ Complete the activities for Chapter 2 in the workbook that accompanies the textbook. Your instructor may use these activities as assignments.

Key Terms

The following terms and those defined in Chapter 2 are important to your understanding of this unit.

delusions	— Inaccurate and unreasonable beliefs that often result in decision-making errors.
EEG (electro-encephalograph)	— A device that measures the brain's electrical activity.
PET scan (positron emission tomography)	— A computerized radiographic technique that enables physicians to detect metabolic activity of various organs, including the brain.
stigma	— A perceived disgrace.

Video Viewing Questions

1. What are the characteristics of a psychologically healthy person?

2. What are the primary causes of mental disorders? What are typical symptoms of depression? How can one tell if an unhappy person is depressed or simply experiencing normal mood changes?

3. Dr. Leuchter states, "The major struggle that we face in psychiatry is…overcoming the stigmas associated with mental illness." What does he mean?

4. What are the typical symptoms of schizophrenia?

5. What treatments are available to help people with psychological disorders? Are these treatments safe and effective?

6. What are the differences between anorexia nervosa and bulimia nervosa? Who is most at risk of developing these conditions? How are these disorders treated?

Self-Test

Multiple Choice

1. Which of the following statements about mentally healthy people is *not* true?
   a. Mentally healthy people engage the world in a meaningful manner.
   b. Mentally healthy people suffer from depression, mania and compulsions, but they are able to conceal their abnormal feelings.
   c. Mentally healthy people are able to enjoy life.
   d. Mentally healthy people are productive and feel successful.

2. Katie is severely depressed. Although medications are available that could treat her depression, she refuses to see a physician for an evaluation of her psychological status. According to Dr. Leuchter, why do people like Katie avoid getting help for their psychological problems?
    a. Today, most depressed people are too busy to have a physician's psychiatric evaluation.
    b. Since most antidepressant medications have serious side effects, depressed people try to feel better without taking them.
    c. In our society, a stigma is associated with having mental illnesses such as depression.
    d. People suffering from depression enjoy the sympathetic attention they receive from others.

3. Which of the following conditions does not increase the risk of psychiatric disorders?
    a. Living in coastal regions.
    b. Injuring certain parts of the brain.
    c. Having a first degree relative with a psychiatric disorder.
    d. Facing difficult life events.

4. Jeanne thinks her 18-year old son is suffering from depression. Which of the following conditions is a common symptom of this psychological disorder?
    a. Dementia
    b. Incontinence
    c. Loss of energy
    d. Elevated mood

5. Which of the following conditions is *not* a cause of dementia?
    a. Brain injuries
    b. Osteoporosis
    c. Aging
    d. Brain tumors

6. Lisa Beth thinks she is Cleopatra, the queen of ancient Egypt. She tells people that her three cats are her "servants." She gives orders to her "servants" and claims to hear them speak to her in Egyptian. Lisa Beth is probably suffering from
    a. depression.
    b. anxiety.
    c. schizophrenia.
    d. bipolar disorder.

7. Based on what you have learned from watching "State of Mind," which of the following statements is correct?
    a. Depressed people typically hide their true feelings by being sociable, friendly, and happy.
    b. The brain and body of a depressed person undergo chemical changes that prevent the person from being himself or herself.
    c. Eating disorders such as anorexia nervosa and bulimia nervosa primarily affect young men.
    d. Unfortunately, most antidepressant medications have unpleasant side effects that limit their usefulness.

8. Specialists who treat psychological problems often recommend
   a. psychotherapy.
   b. electrotherapy.
   c. radiotherapy.
   d. magnetotherapy.

9. People who are suffering from anorexia nervosa and bulimia nervosa have a morbid fear of
   a. sugar.
   b. alcohol.
   c. fat.
   d. depression.

10. Tracy's body weight is normal. Her friends are amazed at the huge amounts of cookies, chips, and pizza she can eat at one time without gaining weight. After she eats the food, she excuses herself to go to the bathroom. Her friends don't know that she is depressed and worried about gaining weight. Tracy is probably suffering from
    a. intestinal tapeworms.
    b. stomach parasites.
    c. hyperthyroidism.
    d. bulimia nervosa.

11. Young people who have a high risk of eating disorders tend to exhibit a cluster of certain character traits. For example, a young woman who is at risk of anorexia nervosa is likely to be
    a. obese.
    b. insecure.
    c. rebellious.
    d. assertive.

12. According to Dr. Strober, _____ may be the only event that triggers the development of an eating disorder.
    a. death of a close relative
    b. graduation from high school
    c. breaking up with a boyfriend
    d. going through puberty

Short Answer

13. Explain how one can distinguish between a person who is psychologically healthy and one who is not.

14. Mental illnesses are complex disorders; in many instances, it is difficult to determine causation. Discuss biological and environmental factors that can result in mental illness.

15. People with anorexia nervosa and bulimia nervosa have similar attitudes concerning body image. Additionally, certain underlying psychological disturbances are associated with these disorders. Compare anorexia nervosa and bulimia nervosa. Discuss the similarities and differences between these two eating disorders.

Expanded Analysis

1. Dr. Leuchter says, "Obviously depressed mood is the most common manifestation of depression...[other manifestations include] loss of energy, difficulty functioning on the job, feeling like you can't cope...feeling like you just want to withdraw and do nothing." From time to time you have probably had these feelings. How can you tell if your feelings were normal "ups and downs" or signs on depression?

2. Girls who have certain personality traits are prone to eating disorders, especially when they reach puberty. Boys and young men, however, rarely develop these conditions. What role does society play in the development of eating disorders, especially among teenage girls?

3. The stigma associated with mental illness prevents many people with these disorders from seeking treatment. What do you think can be done to reduce the stigma associated with having a psychological disturbance?

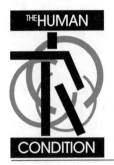

THE HUMAN
CONDITION

4

Lives in Balance

Learning Objectives

Upon completing this lesson, you should be familiar with the facts and concepts presented in the lesson and should be able to:

○ Discuss the physical and psychological effects of chronic stress.

○ Differentiate between "productive" and "non-productive" stress.

○ Name three characteristics of people with "hardy" personalities.

○ Describe the emotional responses that people often experience after life-threatening events.

○ Give examples of effective stress-reduction techniques; apply at least one of these techniques to a stressful situation you may experience.

Overview

Regardless of age, nearly everyone experiences stress each day. Some stress is necessary and beneficial because it provides opportunities for personal growth. Everyday stressors, however, can produce physical and emotional effects that accumulate over time and become harmful to our health and well-being. The "stressed-out" person feels tense, anxious, and unable to concentrate, work, or function socially.

Some people can handle stress better than others. What makes these individuals better able to cope with stress? According to Dr. Khoshaba, Director of Program Development and Training at the Hardiness Institute in Newport Beach, California, *hardiness* is "the ability to transform the problems [people] encounter in life in a way that enhances their performance, their morale, their conduct, and their health." Hardy people accept change as an aspect of living and have positive problem-solving skills. People who resist change and feel that "bad things" should not happen to them are more likely to have problems managing stress.

Dr. Salvatore Maddi, President of The Hardiness Institute, notes that hardiness is a "... personality pattern where you have certain attitudes, certain skills; a sense of commitment, a sense of control, and a sense of challenge." A person can manage stress by developing a plan of action that includes recognizing situations that create obstacles to fulfilling his or her needs. In addition to recognizing stressful situations, many stress management plans include some form of "quiet time," such as prayer or meditation.

Catastrophic Events

Occasionally individuals experience extremely stressful, even life-threatening situations such as a natural disaster, war, or a homicidal attack. Typically, survivors of these incidents suffer from post-traumatic stress disorder (PTSD). PTSD is a chronic condition characterized by distressing psychological symptoms such as unwanted recollections and flashbacks of the terrible events. After the critical incident, victims may receive psychological counseling to help them cope, but they must live with the memory of the terrifying experience for the rest of their lives.

Nancy Bohl, PhD, Director of The Counseling Team of San Bernardino, California, describes the emotional stages that survivors of catastrophic life events typically experience. These stages include denial, anger, and acceptance. In 1998, Dr. Bohl counseled the victims of a gunman's attack on Riverside, California's city council members. The council members' dramatic recollections of the event and their coping responses are highlighted in "Lives in Balance."

Assignments

◯ Read Chapter 3, "Stress and Its Management," and review the section on post-traumatic stress disorder, page 38, in Chapter 2 of Alters & Schiff, *Essential Concepts for Healthy Living*, 4th edition. You may find it helpful to take notes on your reading. Then read the Learning Objectives and Overview for this lesson. Review the Key Terms below.

◯ Scan the Video Viewing Questions, and then watch the video program for Lesson 4, "Lives in Balance."

◯ After watching the video, answer the Video Viewing Questions and assess your learning with the Self-Test.

◯ Complete the activities for Chapter 3 in the workbook that accompanies the textbook. Your instructor may use these activities as assignments.

Key Terms

The following term and those defined in Chapter 3 of the textbook are important to your understanding of this unit.

hardiness — Pertaining to stress, a set of attitudes possessed by an individual that helps him or her cope with stress.

Video Viewing Questions

1. Dr. Khoshaba says that you need a certain amount of contrast in experience to grow, a certain amount of conflict facilitates developmental growth, and that stress is necessary to some degree. What does she mean?

2. What is the difference between productive and non-productive stress? How does the body respond physically during the "flight or fight" reaction? According to Dr. Maddi, what are signs of a "behavioral breakdown?"

3. Dr. Nancy Bohl describes the emotional states that victims typically experience after a tragic and life-threatening event. What are these emotional stages? Which stage usually occurs first? Which stage usually occurs last?

4. In October 1998, members of the City Council of Riverside City, California were attacked by a gunman who entered the council's chambers. How did this terrifying experience affect the lives of the victims after the attack?

Self-Test

1. Which of the following physical or emotional changes occur during the "fight or flight" response to stressful situations?

   Multiple Choice

   a. Slowed heart rate
   b. Sleepiness
   c. Anxiousness
   d. Euphoria

2. People who have the _____ personality trait are able to deal with stress effectively.
   a. hardiness
   b. ruthless
   c. ingenious
   d. shyness

3. According to Dr. Maddi, which of the following attitudes is a characteristic of person who handles stress well?
   a. Sense of challenge
   b. Sense of balance
   c. Sense of awareness
   d. Sense of timing

4. Kurt's job is extremely stressful. He is interested in finding some time each day to relax. Which of the following activities would you recommend?
   a. Jogging
   b. Meditation
   c. Playing the piano
   d. Ballroom dancing

5. Three years ago, Ursula's home and the homes of thirty of her neighbors were completely destroyed when a brush fire got out of control. Although her house has been rebuilt, Ursula has nightmares and flashbacks of the night that the fire swept through her community. She keeps reliving the horror of watching her next door neighbor die while trying to get his dog out of his burning house. Ursula is suffering from
   a. catastrophic stress breakdown.
   b. psychotic distress syndrome.
   c. chronic stressful malingering.
   d. post-traumatic stress disorder.

6. After undergoing an extremely traumatic experience, people need to undergo a group process to talk about the incident and release their emotions. Professional counselors call this process
   a. validation.
   b. venting.
   c. debriefing.
   d. reliving.

7. People who survive traumatic events go through various emotional stages. The first emotional stage is
   a. venting.
   b. anger.
   c. denial.
   d. acceptance.

8. In 1996 a hurricane in Florida destroyed Jenna's house. Jenna survived by hiding in a hall closet. Within days of the storm, she received counseling to help her cope with the loss. Two years after the frightening experience, she has been able to move on with her life. She has reached the _____ stage of responding to the stressful event.
   a. venting
   b. anger
   c. denial
   d. acceptance

Short Answer

9. Arthur has a demanding but low-paying job. Recently he began attending night school at a community college because he decided to make a career change. When he comes home from work, he grabs something to eat, plays for a few minutes with his two small children, then leaves for his classes. Everyday seems to bring a new challenge. Nevertheless, Arthur thinks he has an average amount of stress in his life. Explain how Arthur can tell if he is dealing effectively with his stressors?

10. Meg has the hardiness personality trait that enables her to deal with stress effectively. Explain how Meg's attitudes enable her to cope with stress in a positive way.

11. Late in the afternoon on May 3,1999 a series of tornadoes rapidly developed and moved through parts of the Midwest. The twisters killed 46 people, injured hundreds of others, and demolished thousands of homes and businesses. One of the tornadoes tore a path of destruction a half-

mile wide through Oklahoma City. After the storm, people surveyed the damage in disbelief. Discuss the major emotional stages that you would expect the survivors to experience as they recover from the catastrophe.

Expanded Analysis

1. Dr. Maddi describes the characteristics of someone with a hardy personaltiy. Would you consider yourself someone with a hardy personality? Is there anything you think you could do to help you cope with stress better?

2. It seems that as terrible tragedies such as the Columbine, Colorado high school shootings and the Oklahoma City bombing happen, news photographers and reporters are on the scene. Are there any restrictions placed on the media when reporting such events? Do you think media should be prevented from photographing or interviewing victims or survivors at the scene of the incident?

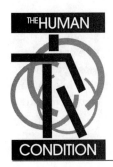

5

Behind Closed Doors

Learning Objectives

Upon completing this lesson, you should be familiar with the facts and concepts presented in this lesson and should be able to:

○ Describe the effects of violence on health and society.

○ Identify and discuss at least three of the root causes of violence and violent behavior.

○ Classify various forms of violence and abuse.

○ Discuss the factors that influence a person's risk of violence.

○ Assess actions that communities and individuals can take to reduce the incidence of violence and their vulnerability to violence.

Overview

Although homicide rates are declining in the United States, violence and abuse are still major public health concerns. Violent behavior occurs on the mean streets of inner cities and in the sprawling homes of wealthy suburbs. It may surprise you to learn that you are more likely to be hurt by someone you know than by a stranger.

Violence is an American epidemic. Like an infectious disease, it spreads throughout a population. Fortunately, immunizations can prevent epidemics of many serious infectious diseases. Is it possible to "immunize" children against the violence epidemic? Some experts think that by understanding the factors that contribute to violence, we may help prevent it.

The origins of violent and abusive behavior are complex, but the accessibility of guns, widespread use of alcohol and other drugs, and poverty are major factors that contribute to the epidemic of violence in the United States. In many low-income communities, youth have few alternatives to joining gangs or engaging in delinquent behavior. The SIMBA Violence Prevention Program in Atlanta, Georgia, is an example of one community's efforts to reduce the likelihood that youth will return to violent behavior when they get out of

Contributing Factors

prison. Teaching violence prevention skills is a major focus of SIMBA instructors.

In the United States, many people experience abuse and violence in their homes. According to Dr. Heger, Director of the Violence Intervention Program at Los Angeles County, USC Medical Center, "Most cases of domestic violence start with emotional violence." Children and adults who live and associate with people who remind them constantly of their inadequacies often develop low self-esteem and can become more easily enraged. Although anger is a normal emotion, it is harmful when not expressed in socially acceptable ways. People need to learn self-respect as well as ways to cope with unpleasant situations that do not involve violence.

Social traditions contribute to the perpetuation of violence. In many cultures, wives are seen as the property of their husbands; therefore, husbands are assumed to have the right to abuse their wives in those societies. Although the belief that wife beating is an acceptable role for husbands is changing in Western cultures, it is still common in other parts of the world. For more information about the mistreatment of women in other countries, read the Diversity in Health Box in Chapter 4 of your textbook.

Children who are witness to, or victims of, parental neglect or domestic abuse are more likely to become neglectful parents or abusive adults in their own homes. Such conditions are not confined to specific racial or ethnic groups or to impoverished households. In the United States, child abuse and neglect are pervasive and occur in affluent as well as poor neighborhoods.

Treating the Epidemic

It is probably unlikely that everyone can learn to settle their disputes without harming themselves or others. However, we can reduce the prevalence of violent and abusive behavior by providing conflict resolution and group counseling programs such as SIMBA. People may be less likely to resort to violence if they understand the sources of their anger and learn socially acceptable coping skills for dealing with the stresses of everyday life. Simple stress management techniques, for example, may help relieve the physical and psychological effects of anger and frustration. As Dr. Heger says, "...violence is not good. It's not okay to hit."

Assignments

◯ Read Chapter 4, "Violence and Abuse," in Alters & Schiff, *Essential Concepts for Healthy Living*, 4th edition. You may find it helpful to take notes on your reading. Then read the Learning Objectives and Overview for this lesson. Review the Key Terms below.

◯ Scan the Video Viewing Questions, and then watch the video program for Lesson 5, "Behind Closed Doors."

◯ After watching the video, answer the Video Viewing Questions and assess your learning with the Self-Test.

◯ Complete the activities for Chapter 4 in the workbook that accompanies the textbook. Your instructor may use these activities as assignments.

Key Terms

The following term and those defined in Chapter 4 are important to your understanding of this unit.

anger management — Learning to direct anger into constructive, rather than negative channels or violence.

stress control — Learning to manage stress through communication and problem solving rather than substance abuse or anger.

Video Viewing Questions

1. Why is violence considered a public health problem? What impact does labeling violence as a public health problem have on communities?

2. Who is at risk of committing violent acts or being a victim of violence? Certain urban areas have high rates of violence. What characteristics of those communities contribute to their high rates of violence? Is violence limited to these areas?

3. Millicent Pierce teaches violence prevention skills to young men who are prone to violence. According to Pierce, what is the number one risk factor? What are other major violence risk factors?

4. According to Dr. Heger, "Most cases of domestic violence start with emotional violence." What are some examples of emotional violence?

5. In discussing domestic violence, Dr. Heger says, "I think society still likes to blame women and children, if they're victims, and likes to find a reason for it." What does she mean?

6. What can an angry individual do to relieve stress? What steps can communities and schools take to reduce the risk of violence?

Self-Test

1. In the United States, the leading cause of death for black adolescents is
   a. automobile accidents.
   b. drug overdoses.
   c. lung cancer.
   d. community violence.

2. For 10 years, Lisa's husband has been beating and verbally abusing her. She doesn't want to leave him because of their two young children. When she complains to her husband's parents, they tell her that if she

Multiple Choice

would just lose a few pounds, cook better meals, or be nicer to her husband that he would stop hurting her. Their response is an example of
a. accepting responsibility.
b. blaming the victim.
c. using inductive reasoning.
d. thinking intuitively.

3. Henry is a 50-year old, unemployed alcoholic who lives with his 85-year-old mother. His mother suffers from severe arthritis and cannot get around the house without using her walker. When Henry needs money, he threatens to harm his mother unless she signs her social security check over to him. Henry's behavior is an example of
a. abuse.
b. neglect.
c. passivity.
d. ignorance.

4. The most common setting for abuse is
a. playgrounds.
b. homes.
c. hospitals.
d. day care facilities.

5. The risk of violence is often related to
a. constructive anger.
b. high self-esteem.
c. gun accessibility.
d. child advocacy.

6. Ten-year old Johnny is unhappy and angry. He is an average student, has poor social skills, and is clumsy. His parents constantly tell him that he is stupid and lazy, and he'll never amount to anything in life if he doesn't do better in school. His classmates harass him and call him "retarded." Even his teachers make him angry by reminding him that his older sister was very smart and a terrific soccer player. According to Dr. Heger in the video "Behind Closed Doors," Johnny is at risk of becoming violent because he is experiencing _____ violence.
a. domestic
b. emotional
c. community
d. peripheral

7. Which of the following statements is true?
a. Conflict resolution programs help youngsters understand that violence is not an acceptable response to stressful situations.
b. Communities with good schools, well-educated residents, and vigilant police forces are immune to violence.
c. Anger is not a healthy emotion, and expressing anger in a relationship has negative effects on everyone.
d. A person is more likely to be attacked by a stranger than someone he or she knows.

Short Answer

8. Discuss factors associated with the risk of juvenile violence. What steps can communities take to reduce the risk of violence among youths?

9. Explain why many public health experts describe violence in America as an "epidemic."

10. Discuss how exposure to domestic violence affects children.

Expanded Analysis

1. Dr. Paul McHugh, Director of the Department of Psychiatry and Behavioral Sciences at Johns Hopkins University Medical School, states, "If violent weapons weren't as accessible, there would be less violence because lots of it occurs impulsively." Explain why you agree or disagree with this statement.

2. A friend of yours says, "I'm glad we live in the suburbs; it's much safer to live here than in the city. You don't have to be afraid of strangers... neighbors know each other." Do you agree or disagree with your friend's statement? Explain why.

3. Why do many people, especially women who are abused by their partners, remain in abusive relationships? What is your community doing to deal with the problem of domestic violence?

4. What would you teach if you were asked to present a conflict resolution program for 5th graders?

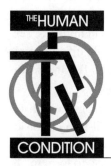

THE HUMAN
CONDITION

6

It's Personal

Learning Objectives

Upon completing this lesson, you should be familiar with the facts and concepts presented in the lesson and should be able to:

○ Recognize that sexuality is an important aspect of human life.

○ Describe factors that influence a person's desire to form intimate relationships.

○ Identify factors that contribute to compatibility.

○ Define homosexuality, heterosexuality, and bisexuality.

○ Explain how culture and society influence sexual behavior.

○ Describe factors that are associated with long-term loving relationships.

Overview

Humans are sexual beings; sexuality affects one's identity, self-esteem, emotions, personality, relationships, and health. Indeed, sexuality influences every aspect of human life.

Being knowledgeable about sexuality is important for maintaining good health and well-being. Many Americans, however, are ignorant about their sexuality and are uncomfortable discussing sexual matters, especially with their young children. Young people, however, are more likely to make responsible decisions concerning their sexuality if they are well informed.

Children want to learn about sexuality, and they want to learn it from their parents. Parents can help by learning more about sex so they can be more comfortable answering their childrens' questions. If children know that their parents are willing to provide reliable information about sex, they are more likely to turn to them for answers to their questions.

People express their sexual behaviors, desires, and attitudes in diverse ways. Sexual orientation is an important and fundamental aspect of a person's sexuality. Although most people are heterosexual, a small percentage of people are homosexual or bisexual.

Sexual Diversity and Relationships

Today most sexologists do not think that homosexuals choose their sexual orientation. Since many homosexuals report that they felt "different" at an early age, scientists suspect there are biological factors than influence sexual orientation. According to Dr. Hamer, researchers have identified genetic markers that code for sexual orientation. Although biological factors are important, the environment also influences sexual orientation.

Regardless of their sexual orientation, people need to establish and maintain satisfying attachments to others for optimal health and well-being. Individuals who have high self esteem, are satisfied with their bodies, are in good health, and have positive feelings about their sexuality are likely to form fulfilling intimate relationships. Although love is difficult to define, people who are in loving relationships share feelings of caring, respect, attachment, commitment, and intimacy.

Assignments

○ Read Chapter 6, "Relationships and Sexuality" in Alters & Schiff, *Essential Concepts for Healthy Living*, 4th edition. You may find it helpful to take notes on your reading. Then read the Learning Objectives and Overview for this lesson. Review the Key Terms below.

○ Scan the Video Viewing Questions, and then watch the video program for Lesson 6, "It's Personal."

○ After watching the video, answer the Video Viewing Questions and assess your learning with the Self-Test.

○ Complete the activities for Chapter 6 in the workbook that accompanies the textbook. Your instructor may use these activities as assignments.

Key Terms

The following terms and those defined in Chapter 6 are important to your understanding of this unit.

bisexual	— A person who engages in sexual activity with people of both sexes.
CDC	— Centers for Disease Control and Prevention
heterosexual	— A person who is sexually attracted to members of the opposite sex.
homophobic	— Pertaining to an intense fear of or hostility toward homosexuals.
homosexual	— A person who is sexually attracted to members of his or her own sex.
sexologist	— A scientist who studies human sexuality (sexology).

Video Viewing Questions

1. How does the typical American attitude toward sex education compare to that of people in the Scandinavian countries? What are the consequences of being sexually ignorant?

2. What information should children learn about sexuality besides the male and female reproductive systems?

3. How diverse are human sexual behavior, preferences, and attitudes?

4. What factors contribute to a person's sexual orientation and which do not? Why is it unlikely that people choose to become homosexuals?

5. What role does one's religious and cultural background play in the development of sexual attitudes and practices?

6. What factors contribute to the formation of healthy relationships?

Self-Test

Multiple Choice

1. Which of the following statements is true?
    a. It is not natural for teenagers to be interested in sex.
    b. In the United States, sexuality is a source of moral, cultural, and political controversy.
    c. Children prefer obtaining sex information from their peers rather than their parents.
    d. Human males tend to have fewer sexual partners than human females.

2. According to Dr. Golden, people in _____ have an enlightened attitude toward sex education.
    a. the United States
    b. Scandinavian countries
    c. Turkey
    d. India

3. As Jeff left a bar that is known to be popular with homosexuals, he was attacked and beaten by a couple of young men who called him "queer" and "faggot." Jeff's attackers are examples of people with
    a. homophilia.
    b. homogenation.
    c. homosaturation.
    d. homophobia.

4. Which of the following statements is true?
    a. Asexuals are people who are interested in having sexual activity with either males or females.
    b. A person who is homophobic wants to have sex only with members of his or her own sex.
    c. There is scientific evidence that links genetic factors with male homosexuality.
    d. The majority of people have a chromosome that is expressed as homosexual behavior.

5. Which of the following factors does *not* appear to contribute to one's sexual orientation?
   a. Environmental factors
   b. Exposure to hormones during fetal development
   c. Genetic expression
   d. Personal choice

6. Which of the following statements is true?
   a. When people are knowledgeable about human sexuality, they are less likely to have unplanned pregnancies.
   b. Studies show that people have the same sexual attitudes and practices, regardless of their religious backgrounds or national origins.
   c. Culture has little influence in the development of sexual attitudes and behaviors.
   d. The first step in forming an emotionally satisfying relationship is establishing sexual intimacy.

7. Which of the following statements is true?
   a. Sexologists are physicians who treat reproductive system disorders.
   b. Sexuality affects a person's identity, self-esteem, emotions, lifestyle, and health.
   c. People only engage in sexual activity for reproductive purposes.
   d. The Kinsey Report is the latest survey of American sexual practices.

Short Answer

8. Explain how you would educate your children about human sexuality. Include the kinds of information about sexuality that you would include.

9. Discuss the social and health consequences of being sexually ignorant.

10. Homosexuals comprise a small percentage of the population. Explain why it seems unlikely that homosexuals "choose" their sexual orientation.

Expanded Analysis

1. A group of people in your school district want to remove the current comprehensive sexual education program from the 8th grade curriculum and replace it with a program that promotes sexual abstinence and fails to provide information about birth control, sexually transmitted infections, or sexual diversity. You have an opportunity to speak before the school board. Prepare a presentation to the school board that would convince its members to keep the current sex education curriculum.

2. The population of the United States is quite diverse. Discuss how a person's cultural, ethnic, and religious backgrounds can influence his or her sexual attitudes and behaviors.

3. In the United States, about one-half of all marriages that take place annually will end in divorce. You have been asked to develop and conduct a program for couples who are planning to marry. The goal of your program is to reduce the likelihood that the couples who participate in the program will get divorced. Develop the pre-marital program; include the kinds of topics about relationships and sexuality that you would cover with the couples.

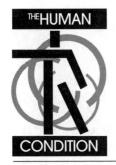

7

Risky Business

Learning Objectives

Upon completing this lesson, you should be familiar with the facts and concepts presented in the lesson and should be able to:

○ Recognize the risks associated with unprotected, casual sex.

○ Compare the advantages and disadvantages of various methods of contraception.

○ Know the signs and symptoms of sexually transmitted diseases, and their long-term effects.

○ Evaluate various approaches that are recommended to prevent, control, and treat sexually transmitted diseases.

Overview

Not every person wants to have a child every time he or she has sex; therefore, responsible people take steps to prevent unwanted pregnancies. Nevertheless, many American couples don't use contraception despite the wide variety of birth control methods that are available. Being unprepared for sexual intercourse may mean having an unwanted pregnancy or contracting a sexually transmitted disease (STD), also referred to as a sexually transmitted infection (STI). Indeed, half of the pregnancies are unwanted or unplanned, and rates of many STDs are rising in the United States.

Most of today's contraceptive methods rely on the woman taking action. Hormonal methods are very effective and reversible but can cause serious side effects. Although female sterilization is an effective way of preventing pregnancy, this method requires surgery and is not easily reversible. Therefore it is important for couples to weigh the risks and benefits before choosing a method of contraception. When contraception is unavailable, abstinence is the safest, most effective way to prevent pregnancy and the transmission of STDs.

In the United States, condoms are a widely available form of birth control, but they are not 100 percent effective as a means of preventing pregnancy and STDs. Health experts recommend combining contraception techniques, such as using condoms and oral contraceptive pills, to reduce the likelihood of STD transmission and pregnancy. (See the section "Protecting Yourself Against STIs" in Chapter 14 of the textbook for information about the use of condoms.)

Sexually Transmitted Diseases

Sexually transmitted diseases are among the most common infectious diseases. Public health officials and medical experts are concerned about rising STD rates in the United States and elsewhere. Viral STDs are especially serious because there are no cures for these diseases, and they can produce serious side effects such as infertility and even death. Dr. Hatcher tells college students, "There are four "H" viruses. You get them...for life. Herpes, Human Papillomavirus, HIV, and Hepatitis B virus."

Human papillomavirus (HPV) is thought to be the most widespread viral STD. Types of this virus are known to cause cervical cancer. Bacterial STDs, such as syphilis, gonorrhea, and chlamydial infections, are also widespread. Gonorrhea and chlamydial infections can cause infertility in women. Although contracting one of these infections is serious, none is as serious as contracting human immunodeficiency virus (HIV), the virus that causes AIDS.

If you have unprotected sex, you can die prematurely from AIDS. At present there is no vaccine to protect against HIV and no cure for AIDS. Many people still think HIV is a disease that only homosexual males contract. Rates of HIV infection, however, are increasing rapidly among women in the United States. People need to realize that HIV is an "equal opportunity virus." Regardless of gender, sexual orientation, socioeconomic status, or level of education, anyone engaging in unprotected sexual intercourse is at risk of contracting HIV. Table 14-1 in your textbook lists characteristics of people who have a high risk of HIV infection.

Although condoms are not fail-safe, the only way to reduce the risk of contracting or spreading HIV is to use condoms during sexual intercourse. Responsible sexual behavior includes taking steps to make sexual intercourse as "safe" as possible.

Assignments

○ Read Chapter 5 "Reproductive Health," and pages 398–415 in Chapter 14, "Infection, Immunity, and Noninfectious Disease." Review "Sexual Response" and "Sexual Dysfunctions," pages 136–139, in Chapter 6 of Alters & Schiff, *Essential Concepts for Healthy Living*, 4th edition. You may find it helpful to take notes on your reading. Then read the Learning Objectives and Overview for this lesson. Review the Key Terms below.

○ Scan the Video Viewing Questions, and then watch the video program for Lesson 7, "Risky Business."

○ After watching the video, answer the Video Viewing Questions and assess your learning with the Self-Test.

○ Complete the activities for Chapters 5 and 14 in the workbook that accompanies the textbook. Your instructor may use these activities as assignments.

Key Terms

The following terms are important to your understanding of this unit.

benign	— Not cancerous.
curettage	— Scraping material from the wall of an organ such as the uterus.
D&C	— Abbreviation for dilatation and curettage, a procedure in which the cervix is dilated to allow an instrument to be inserted so the walls of the uterus can be scraped or suctioned.
hysterectomy	— Surgical removal of the uterus.
progestin	— The female hormone progesterone.
pulmonary embolism	— Something, such as a blood clot, that blocks an artery in the lung.

Video Viewing Questions

1. In the United States, 50 percent of pregnancies are unplanned. What are the effects of teenage pregnancies on young women and their families?

2. About 80 percent of U.S. women use oral contraception (birth control pills) at some time in their lives. Many stop using birth control pills because of side effects. What are the advantages and disadvantages of using oral contraceptives?

3. What are the advantages and disadvantages of Depo-Provera?

4. What can couples do to prevent pregnancy if they have not used contraception during sex or their method of contraception failed?

5. Which form of birth control provides protection against HIV?

6. Dr. Hatcher refers to four "H" sexually transmitted viruses that people get "for life." What are these viruses?

Self-Test

1. Before oral contraceptive pills were introduced, _____ were a popular form of contraception.
   a. abortions
   b. Depo-Provera injections
   c. barrier methods
   d. hysterectomies

Multiple Choice

2. Which of the following statements about oral contraceptive pills is true?
   a. Oral contraceptive pills are not an effective way to control the timing of pregnancy.
   b. Women who use oral contraceptive pills have a lower risk of ovarian cancer than women who do not use oral contraceptives.
   c. Benign breast masses are a common side effect of taking oral contraceptives.
   d. The risk of endometrial cancer increases when taking oral contraceptives.

3. Physicians often prescribe oral contraceptives to women who are over 40 years of age to
   a. produce regular menstrual cycles.
   b. decrease appetite for sweets and fatty foods.
   c. increase circulation.
   d. enhance muscle tone.

4. Theo and Danielle rely on condoms for birth control. Last night the condom slipped off Theo's penis, and semen spilled into Danielle's vagina. What would you suggest as the most effective back up method of contraception for this couple?
   a. Danielle should douche with a carbonated soft drink.
   b. Danielle should take post-coital contraception.
   c. Danielle should have an IUD inserted.
   d. Danielle can do nothing to prevent pregnancy under the circumstances.

5. Which of the following contraception methods is the safest and most effective?
   a. Abstinence
   b. Sterilization
   c. IUD
   d. Oral contraceptive pills

6. Which of the following diseases is a sexually transmitted disease?
   a. Measles
   b. Chlamydia
   c. Cystic fibrosis
   d. Sickle cell anemia

7. If it is untreated, which of the following STDs can result in pelvic inflammatory disease?
   a. Hepatitis B
   b. Herpes
   c. Gonorrhea
   d. AIDS

Matching

Match the form of contraception with the best description that follows.
   a. Depo-Provera
   b. IUD
   c. condom
   d. sterilization

_____ 8. Contraceptive effects are difficult to reverse

36

_____ 9. Protects against HIV

_____ 10. Requires hormonal injections every three months

11. Discuss the health effects of using oral contraceptives for birth control.

Short Answer

12. Your 16-year old son has been going out with the same girl for several weeks and is very attracted to her. You are concerned that his relationship with her will become intimate soon. Discuss what you will tell him to do to avoid becoming a father or getting a sexually transmitted disease.

Expanded Analysis

1. Today's couples have many choices for birth control. In the United States, however, about 50 percent of pregnancies are unintentional. Discuss why many sexually active people do not use contraception.

2. Although few women use the IUD in the United States, this method of contraception is very popular in less developed nations. What factors influence the popularity of a method of contraception?

3. If you had to design the perfect form of contraception, what features would the method have?

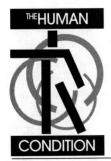

8

The Code

Learning Objectives

Upon completing this lesson, you should be familiar with the facts and concepts presented in the lesson and should be able to:

○ Describe, in general terms, the genetic inheritance each of us receives from our parents and what influence this has on physical appearance, intelligence, behavior and personality, and health.

○ Recognize the goals of the Human Genome Project and its potential to affect personal health.

○ Explain the value of genetic testing and counseling, and the couples who would benefit most from it.

○ Differentiate between *in utero* and newborn health screening tests, and what they are designed to achieve.

○ Examine issues related to genetic modification, and formulate an opinion what, if any, limits should be placed on it.

Overview

Viruses, bacteria, and other pathogens are not responsible for every disease that affects people. Many health conditions are the result of damaged genes (mutations) that are passed down from parents to their children. Genes are pieces of DNA. All the information a living thing needs to develop, function, and maintain itself is coded in the DNA. Not everything about you is preprogrammed in your genes; your environment also plays an important role in determining who you are.

Since 1990, scientists with the Human Genome Project have been determining the sequence of genes in human DNA. According to Dr. Edward McCabe, Chief of Mattel Children's Hospital at the University of California–Los Angeles, "…the goal is to…identify genes and quickly be able to identify mutations." Mutated genes often result in the production of metabolic errors that cause illness and death. By identifying the sequence of each gene, medical researchers can determine if an individual has inherited serious health conditions such as Huntington's disease, cystic fibrosis, Duchenne muscular dystrophy, and certain cancers.

It is possible to test a fetus *in utero* to determine if it carries defective genes. Prenatal testing procedures, such as amniocentesis, are an option for older couples or couples who already have given birth to a child with a serious genetic disorder. If testing results indicate that the fetus has defective genes, the parents may choose to continue or terminate the pregnancy. In a few instances, therapies to correct defects, including fetal surgery *in utero,* can be performed, but such operations are still experimental. After birth, newborns routinely undergo screening for a few conditions such as PKU.

In the future, it will be possible to test the DNA in an egg, a sperm, or an embryo for defective genes. As a result, parents will know in advance which inherited conditions are likely to affect their children, and they will be able to take steps to prevent the conditions from occurring. For example, medical researchers one day may be able to replace defective genes with normal ones, either before fertilization occurs or early in embryonic development.

However, many medical professionals are uncertain about whether this type of gene manipulation is a good idea. According to Alex Capron, the key question with this kind of genetic manipulation is "Where do we stop?" Do we allow doctors to make any and all changes in the interest of creating a better human being, or do we stop at just correcting those conditions that are defined as diseases? In the end, who will determine which genes are manipulated?

Of course, just the capability to detect defective genes in humans creates a number of complex ethical questions that we as a society will be forced to address, even when there is no chance to correct the defects. As Dr. Harold Varmus, the former Director of the National Institutes of Health points out, "Hand in hand with the challenge of using genetic information comes a societal challenge for all of us...to insure that we protect peoples' privacy and...protect them against [the] discrimination...that's likely to occur."

Despite the challenges, determining the sequence of genes in human DNA represents a monumental accomplishment for the scientific community. Within a few years, the public will begin to see benefits from this research. For those who are concerned about the risk of transmitting genetic disorders to their descendants, the future looks much brighter.

Assignments

○ Read pages 379–384 and 413–415 in Chapter 14, "Infection, Immunity, and Noninfectious Disease," of Alters & Schiff, *Essential Concepts for Healthy Living,* 4th edition. You may find it helpful to take notes on your reading. Then read the Learning Objectives and Overview for this lesson. Review the Key Terms below.

○ Scan the Video Viewing Questions, and then watch the video program for Lesson 8, "The Code."

○ After watching the video, answer the Video Viewing Questions and assess your learning with the Self-Test.

○ If you haven't done so already, complete Chapter 14 in the workbook that accompanies the textbook. Your instructor may use these activities as assignments.

Key Terms

The following terms are important to your understanding of this unit.

chromosome — Strand of DNA located in the nucleus of cells that contains genes.

genes — Hereditary material; pieces of DNA that code for the production of certain proteins.

genome — A complete set of chromosomes.

in utero — In the uterus.

mutation — A change in a gene or chromosome.

neural tube — The embryonic structure that develops into the brain and spinal cord.

PKU (phenylketonuria)— An inherited metabolic disease that causes severe mental retardation if the affected newborn is not treated soon after birth.

Video Viewing Questions

1. What is a gene? Where are genes located within cells?

2. What factors influence one's health besides heredity?

3. What is the goal of the Human Genome Project? Approximately how many genes does a human have?

4. What are the benefits of having genetic information? How can genetic information be misused? Do people generally want to know if they have a genetic disorder?

5. What is the purpose of prenatal genetic testing? What choices can parents make when they learn that their fetus carries defective genes? What are *in utero* therapies?

6. In the United States, newborns are routinely screened for certain metabolic conditions and other disorders. What is PKU? What is the value of diagnosing this and other health problems early in infancy?

Self-Test

Multiple Choice

1. Genes are
   a. portions of cytochromes.
   b. fragments of cholesterol.
   c. parts of cell membranes.
   d. pieces of DNA.

2. If you wanted to sequence a person's genes, where would you find them?
   a. In DNA
   b. In chromosomes
   c. In SIDS
   d. In PKU

3. Which of the following statements is true?
   a. The goal of the Human Genome Project was to sequence an entire set of human genes.
   b. The nucleus of a human cell contains approximately 10,000 genes and their variants.
   c. Genes determine everything about a person, including his or her physical traits, personality, and reactions to situations.
   d. By 1999, scientists concluded that it was impossible to sequence the human genome.

4. Environmental factors, such as exposure to x-rays or toxic chemicals, can damage genes. A damaged gene is a
   a. clone.
   b. mutation.
   c. deletion.
   d. chromosome.

5. Katherine is 30 years old. Her father was healthy until he was in his early forties. At that time, he developed a rare neurological disease that eventually killed him. Katherine can have genetic testing to determine if she will develop this late-onset hereditary condition. The condition she may have inherited from her father is
   a. cystic fibrosis.
   b. sickle cell anemia.
   c. malaria.
   d. Huntington's disease.

6. Which of the following conditions is an inherited disorder that causes severe mental retardation if a special diet is not maintained after birth?
   a. Huntington's disease
   b. Sickle cell anemia
   c. PKU
   d. Cystic fibrosis

7. Alex and his wife are healthy, but their first child was born with cystic fibrosis, a recessive genetic disorder. Therefore, Alex and his wife are _____ of the defective gene that results in cystic fibrosis.
   a. clones
   b. carriers
   c. genomes
   d. chromatids

8. Carmen was 7 months pregnant when her physician determined that her unborn fetus had a neural tube defect. What might be done to treat the defect before the fetus is born?

    a. Chemotherapy

    b. Gene therapy

    c. *In utero* therapy

    d. Nothing can be done to treat the defect before birth.

9. Testing for PKU is a form of _____ testing.

    a. chromosomal

    b. newborn

    c. *in utero*

    d. *in vitro*

Short Answer

10. Dr. Paul McHugh, the Director of Department of Psychiatry and Behavioral Sciences and Psychiatrist-in-Chief at Johns Hopkins University Hospital, says, "Genes are just DNA. They aren't destiny." Explain which characteristics are determined almost entirely by genes and which are influenced in part by environmental conditions.

11. Discuss the pros and cons of obtaining genetic information concerning your health status.

12. Discuss the value of prenatal screening.

Expanded Analysis

1. For parents who carry genes for serious defects or diseases, genetic manipulation provides an opportunity to avoid passing down these genes to their offspring. Nevertheless, Alex Capron, co-director of the Pacific Center for Health Policy and Ethics at the University of Southern California, raises some serious ethical questions concerning such technology. Capron says, "…as we get to this kind of genetic manipulation…where do we stop? Do we stop only in correcting things that are identified as a disease, and then how do we decide and who decides what a disease is? Or do we [make any changes] including adding greater capabilities, making a person perform at the highest human level, or even going beyond that?" Discuss potential dangers of genetic manipulation.

2. If a genetic disorder occurs in your family and scientists have a DNA test to detect the defective genes, would you want to know if you have inherited the disorder? Explain why you would or would not want to have the testing.

3. As in the case of the Merten family, signs of child abuse can actually be the result of an undiagnosed genetic disorder. What could hospital emergency room personnel do to avoid making false accusations of child abuse in these rare situations?

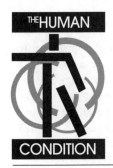

9

Haley or Matthew's Story

Learning Objectives

Upon completing this lesson, you should be familiar with the facts and concepts presented in the lesson and should be able to:

○ Discuss actions that a woman can take to increase her chances of having a successful pregnancy and a healthy baby.

○ Identify major causes of infertility and discuss what can be done to help infertile couples become pregnant.

○ Recognize factors related to premature birth, and the health difficulties a child may experience as a result of an extremely early, pre-term birth.

○ Describe the events that occur at each stage of the birth process.

○ Give examples of the benefits of breast-feeding.

Overview

During pregnancy, a woman's body undergoes numerous changes as it nurtures and protects the developing fetus. When planning a pregnancy, a woman should seek health information and advice from a health care practitioner. After becoming pregnant, she should obtain prenatal care and follow a healthy lifestyle that includes eating a proper diet; avoiding alcohol, tobacco, and other drugs; exercising regularly; and managing stress. These steps can increase the likelihood that her baby will have a healthy start in life.

Unfortunately, not every woman plans to become pregnant or follows a healthy lifestyle during this time of her life. Many women, for example, are not aware of or simply ignore public health warnings about the dangers of smoking cigarettes and drinking alcohol during pregnancy. Other mothers-to-be eat nutritionally inadequate diets. As a result, their pregnancies have a high risk of ending in miscarriage or premature birth. Babies who are born too early are more likely to be underweight, develop breathing problems, suffer brain damage, and die during the first year of life than babies who are full-term. By beginning prenatal care early in her pregnancy, a woman increases her chances of having a healthy full-term infant. As Dr. Sola notes, "...if there is a lack of prenatal care, there is a high incidence of prematurity."

Infertility

Overcoming infertility is often a frustrating experience for those who want to become pregnant. The most frequent causes of infertility are a low sperm count, failure to ovulate, and blockages of the reproductive tract. Age also influences fertility; as a woman grows older, her fertility declines. Additionally, psychological stress can reduce the fertility of a woman, especially a woman who is over 30 years of age. If physicians can pinpoint the cause of a couple's infertility, they often can treat the condition. Nevertheless, many couples still are unable to conceive after receiving treatment for infertility.

Life after Birth

In the past, newborns were taken away from their mothers immediately after birth and placed in a nursery to avoid infections. Today, health care practitioners recognize the importance of early bonding between mother and child. Physicians usually allow new mothers to spend time with their babies soon after birth. This practice gives the mother a chance to get to know her baby and begin the process of becoming emotionally attached to the child.

Many women choose to breast feed their babies. The results of numerous scientific studies indicate that breast-fed babies have fewer respiratory and intestinal infections than formula-fed babies.

Assignments

O Review the "Pregnancy and Human Development" section of Chapter 5, pages 102–112, in Alters & Schiff, *Essential Concepts for Healthy Living*, 4th edition. For more information about breast-feeding, read the "Across the Lifespan" section of Chapter 9, pages 248–251. You may find it helpful to take notes on your reading. Then read the Learning Objectives and Overview for this lesson. Review the Key Terms below.

O Scan the Video Viewing Questions, and then watch the video program for Lesson 9, "Haley or Matthew's Story."

O After watching the video, answer the Video Viewing Questions and assess your learning with the Self-Test.

O Complete the activities for Chapter 5 in the workbook that accompanies the textbook. Your instructor may use these activities as assignments.

Key Terms

The following terms and those in Chapter 5 of your textbook are important to your understanding of this unit.

amniocentesis — A prenatal screening procedure in which a small amount of amniotic fluid that surrounds the fetus is removed. Fetal cells in the fluid are analyzed to discover genetic abnormalities.

antisepsis	— Destruction of disease-causing microorganisms to prevent infections.
folic acid	— A B-vitamin.
neural tube	— The embryonic structure that develops into the brain and spinal cord.
pre-term	— Premature; fetus is less than 38 weeks of age and weighs less than 5 pounds.
spina bifida	— A birth defect in which some of the spinal bones do not close around the spinal cord. As a result, a section of spinal cord protrudes from the infant's back.
ultrasound	— A prenatal screening procedure that uses sound waves to provide physical information about a fetus.

Video Viewing Questions

1. What can women do to plan for pregnancy? How can the mother's use of drugs such as alcohol and tobacco affect an embryo/fetus? Which group of American women is not heeding warnings about drinking alcoholic beverages during pregnancy? How does smoking affect the outcome of pregnancy?

2. Although a pregnant woman is not "eating for two," proper nutrition is very important during pregnancy. What are the possible consequences of poor eating habits during pregnancy?

3. What factors may contribute to premature birth? What serious problems often affect premature infants, especially those weighing less than three pounds?

4. What are the benefits of breast-feeding a baby?

Self-Test

1. Approximately _____ of women plan their pregnancies and could receive pre-pregnancy counseling.
   a. one-half
   b. one-third
   c. one-fourth
   d. one-fifth

2. Which of the following statements is true?
   a. Taking amino acids for at least a month before pregnancy can prevent neural tube defects from developing in the embryo.
   b. Most health experts agree that a pregnant woman can have 1 to 2 alcoholic drinks without harming her embryo/fetus.

Multiple Choice

47

c. A pregnant woman who abuses an addictive drug regularly can give birth to a baby who is addicted to the drug.

    d. Low-income American women drink five times more alcohol during pregnancy than well-educated, wealthy women.

3. Pregnant women who _____ have an increased risk of delivering a low birth-weight baby who is weak and vulnerable to illness.
    a. drink 8 glasses of water daily
    b. take folic acid supplements
    c. smoke cigarettes
    d. eat red meats

4. Compared to babies of non-smoking mothers, babies of mothers who smoked during pregnancy have a higher risk of dying from
    a. Hurler's syndrome.
    b. acquired immunodeficiency syndrome.
    c. fetal nicotine toxicity syndrome.
    d. sudden infant death syndrome.

5. Women who skip meals and fast during pregnancy have a high risk of
    a. bulimia nervosa.
    b. fetal obesity.
    c. miscarriage.
    d. PKU.

6. According to Dr. Hobel, women who experience stress early in their pregnancies have a greater risk of
    a. miscarriage.
    b. Hurler's syndrome.
    c. gallbladder cancer.
    d. periodontal disease.

7. In the United States, _____ is associated with a high risk of premature birth.
    a. driving small cars
    b. exercising regularly
    c. failing to obtain prenatal care
    d. living in suburban areas

8. Pre-term babies, especially ones that weigh less than 3 pounds, require intensive newborn medical care. These babies have a high risk of
    a. obesity.
    b. breathing problems.
    c. PKU.
    d. dystic fibrosis.

9. Which of the following statements is *not* true?
    a. Pre-term babies are more likely to have cerebral palsy and mental retardation than full term babies.
    b. Babies who weigh less than 3 pounds at birth must have intensive medical care to survive.
    c. In the United States, about one-third of babies are born prematurely.
    d. Pregnant women who receive prenatal care are more likely to deliver healthy full-term babies than those who do not receive prenatal care.

10. A major cause of *male* infertility is
    a. old eggs.
    b. psychosocial stress.
    c. blocked oviducts.
    d. low sperm count.

11. Which of the following prenatal screening procedures uses high frequency sound waves to visualize a fetus?
    a. ultrasound
    b. amniocentesis
    c. fetal sonar monitoring
    d. intrauterine microwaves

12. Kim is having difficulty breast feeding her new baby. She can't turn to her mother or friends for advice because they didn't breast-feed their children. The _____ is the best source of support and answers to Kim's breast-feeding questions.
    a. La Leche League
    b. local health department
    c. local pharmacist
    d. FDA

Short Answer

13. Cindy is 4 months pregnant. To avoid gaining too much weight during pregnancy, she skips breakfast and doesn't eat anything after dinner. Discuss the effects that Cindy's eating habits may have on her pregnancy. What advice would you give to Cindy?

14. After a year of trying, Omar and Catlin have been unable to conceive. They have decided to have an infertility expert determine why Catlin has been unable to become pregnant. Explain what factors could be responsible for the couple's infertility.

15. A friend of yours is pregnant. She asks you if she should breast-feed her baby. Discuss what you would tell her.

Expanded Analysis

1. Scientific studies do not support the popular belief that reading Shakespeare aloud or listening to classical music during pregnancy increases the intelligence of the fetus. Explain how these activities might nonetheless benefit the health of a pregnant woman.

2. You have been asked to develop a public health campaign to encourage young women to plan their pregnancies and obtain pre-pregnancy counseling. Discuss the basic goals of your campaign and how you would reach this population of women before they become pregnant.

3. In the early 1900s, babies who were born in hospitals were whisked away to a nursery after birth. What was the rationale for keeping newborns separated from their mothers? Today, healthy newborns are given more time with their mothers. Discuss the advantages of allowing mothers to be with their infants immediately after they are born.

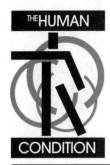

10

The Growing Years

Learning Objectives

Upon completing this lesson, you should be familiar with the facts, terms, and concepts presented in the lesson and should be able to:

○ Recognize that health habits formed in childhood influence the health profile of the adult.

○ Evaluate the significance of vaccinations, of limited exposure to the "outside world," of reading and other forms of stimulation during the first year of a child's life.

○ Identify sources of accidents and injury to toddlers and children, and the steps caregivers can take to protect young ones.

○ Create a list of strategies that can help children develop healthy eating habits, as well as approaches that should be avoided.

○ Differentiate between healthy and stressful levels of activity for children and families.

○ Describe challenges to the health of adolescents, particularly in inner city areas.

Overview

You may have heard the saying "children are our most precious resource." Like other natural resources, children need to be protected and nurtured because of the important role they will have in society in the future. Most parents, however, find it challenging to raise healthy children in today's often-perilous world. Providing food, shelter, and clothing for a child is not enough. Parents and other caretakers must also meet a child's need for an environment that fosters their normal intellectual and emotional development. Many children spend the first years of their lives in daycare settings that meet the youngsters' basic needs, but often fail to provide enough physical and intellectual stimulation.

As children grow and become more independent, they need freedom to play in and explore their environment, but they are often unable to recognize hazardous conditions. Unintentional injuries (accidents) are the major health threat to children over one year of age. Most deaths from such injuries are preventable, such as deaths due to motor vehicle crashes, drowning, and house fires. Sadly, many children also die as the result of violence in their homes or neighborhoods. It is the responsibility of a child's caretakers to make sure the child's environment is as safe as possible and to teach the child basic safety principles.

Long-term Health Concerns

It may be difficult to believe, but obese children are suffering from malnutrition. According to Dr. Barbara Korsch, a pediatrician at Children's Hospital, Los Angeles, "Now our biggest, biggest problem, 'big' in every sense of the word, is obesity at all ages." Childhood obesity is associated with type II diabetes as well as elevated blood cholesterol and blood pressure levels. Obese children are likely to remain overweight as they mature, and being overweight increases the risk of heart disease in middle age. Heart disease is the number one killer of adult Americans.

As with adults, poor eating habits and a lack of physical activity play major roles in the development of excess body fat in children. Many children spend too much time in passive activities such as watching television and not enough time in physically demanding activities such as playing basketball outdoors. Many children in urban areas, however, live in unsafe neighborhoods, so parents may not encourage their children to go outdoors and play. In these instances, parents may have to find alternative places for children to be physically active while under adult supervision, such as walking in malls or through public places such as zoos or parks.

Seeking Advice

Adolescence is a time when youngsters establish behaviors that may last a lifetime and when experimentation with risky behaviors usually begins. Unintentional injuries, homicide, and suicide are major causes of death for American teenagers, and alcohol abuse, pregnancy, and sexually transmitted infections are national problems.

By the time children reach puberty, they should recognize that a personal physician provides preventive care and treats a variety of physical ailments. Teenagers need to know that physicians also can provide help for their psychological problems. Many youngsters are afraid to discuss their personal concerns with parents, and their parents often do not have the time to communicate with them. If teens have developed a trusting relationship with their physicians, they may be more willing to seek help and information from these health care experts.

Whether it's obtaining adequate preventive care for a child, teaching a child safe behaviors, or preparing nutritious meals, parents should take an active role in protecting their children's health. Parents can accomplish this role by taking the time to talk with their children, serving as a primary source of information and modeling healthy lifestyles.

Assignments

○ Read the Learning Objectives and Overview for this lesson. Review the Key Terms below.

○ Scan the Video Viewing Questions, and then watch the video program for Lesson 10, "The Growing Years."

○ After watching the video, answer the Video Viewing Questions and assess your learning with the Self-Test.

Key Terms

The following terms are important to your understanding of this unit.

H-flu	— Nickname for Haemophilus type b, a type of bacteria that causes a common infection that can result in pneumonia or meningitis.
neophobia	— Fear of new things, such as new foods.
otitis media	— Middle ear infections.

Video Viewing Questions

1. In the last half of the twentieth century, immunizations dramatically reduced the risk of childhood infections such as measles, mumps, and polio, as well as the meningitis caused by Haemophilus type B bacteria. Why are respiratory and middle ear infections still common among young children?

2. Although infants need to be kept warm, fed, and have their diapers changed, they also need to be touched, held, and stimulated intellectually. What can happen to an infant who is deprived of such stimulation? What are some of the benefits of the Reach Out and Read program?

3. Why are children at risk of suffering unintentional injuries? What role should caretakers play in preventing such injuries to children?

4. Which toys and activities are appropriate for young children?

5. How can parents and caretakers be positive role models for children?

6. Adolescents need to confide in trustworthy adults who also serve as sources of information and advice. Who would be good choices for this role?

Self-Test

Multiple Choice

1. According to Dr. Korsch, which of the following infections is very common among young children?
   a. Polio
   b. Measles
   c. Otitis media
   d. Pneumonia

2. Molly is three years old. Her parents made sure that she is up-to-date with her childhood immunizations. Molly has protection against which of the following infectious diseases?
   a. Scarlet fever
   b. Botulism
   c. Mumps
   d. Hepatitis B

3. Which of the following conditions enhances the development of neural connections in an infant's brain?
   a. Exposing the child to cigarette smoke
   b. Reading picture books to the child
   c. Changing the child's diapers regularly
   d. Keeping the child reasonably warm

4. The major cause of preventable death in children is
   a. exposure to cigarette smoke.
   b. unintended injuries.
   c. cystic fibrosis.
   d. arterial plaques.

5. In the United States, _____ is a major cause of injury to children.
   a. gun violence
   b. medical malpractice
   c. drug overdose
   d. food poisoning

6. You would like to buy a gift for your cousin's new baby. Which of the following gifts is not recommended for babies because it is unsafe?
   a. Plastic teething ring
   b. Picture book
   c. Baby walker
   d. Cotton blanket

7. The dramatic rise in the prevalence of childhood obesity has resulted in an increase in cases of _____ in this population.
   a. rheumatic fever
   b. otitis media
   c. Type II diabetes
   d. congenital porphyria

8. Jared is having some problems adjusting to middle school. He does not feel comfortable talking to his parents about his feelings or about drugs because they are so judgmental. Furthermore, he is concerned about

some of the physical changes that are happening to his body as he enters puberty. Who would you recommend as a reliable and trustworthy source of information for Jared?

a. Jared's girlfriend's parents
b. Jared's personal physician
c. Jared's grandparents
d. Jared's best friend

9. A friend has a 7-year old child who weighs 20 pounds more than what is considered healthy for his height. Your friend asks for your advice to help the child lose weight safely. Which of the following recommendations would you make?
   a. Remove all sugary and fatty foods from the child's diet.
   b. Ask the child's doctor to prescribe diet pills that are safe for children.
   c. Allow the child to have moderate amounts of fattening foods and encourage him to be more physically active.
   d. Don't worry about the child's weight because he'll outgrow it.

10. Which of the following statements is true?
    a. Most young children are willing to eat new foods when they are served.
    b. Children who live in cities are more likely to play outdoors than children in rural areas.
    c. Children who take drugs have a high risk of being involved in violent acts.
    d. Adolescent boys and girls have similar fitness and physical activity levels.

Short Answer

11. Discuss why the percentage of obese children increased dramatically in the United States during the past 25 years.

12. When you think of being a child, you probably think of carefree days and playing with friends. Explain why it is important for children to be physically active.

13. Many parents don't have the time to read picture books to their children. Why is this activity important?

Expanded Analysis

1. Some parents are so concerned about the possible rare but serious side effects associated with routine immunization during childhood that they refuse to have their children vaccinated. What are the risks of childhood immunizations? In the United States, how many children develop serious side effects as a result of being immunized? Do you think the benefits of immunizations outweigh the risks?

2. In the United States, how serious is the problem of children using guns to injure or kill themselves or others? When children use guns to cause such harm, should the owners of the guns be held responsible?

3. If food should not be used as a reward for a child's good behavior, what non-food awards can be substituted?

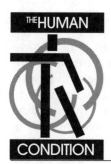

THE HUMAN
CONDITION

11

Web of Addiction

Learning Objectives

Upon completing this lesson, you should be familiar with the facts, terms, and concepts presented in this lesson and should be able to:

O Recognize the pervasiveness of drug abuse across all sectors of society, and the genetic and environmental factors that contribute to it.

O Compare the effects of major psychoactive drugs on the human body.

O Recognize the social and personal costs of drug addiction.

O Describe treatment strategies for drug addiction.

O Explain why many people find it difficult to stay substance free.

Overview

Drug addiction is a disease that has reached epidemic proportions in the United States. "Drug addiction is...[a] horrible, sneaky, life destroying, family destroying illness," says Sandra McDonald, director of a community organization in Atlanta that provides treatment and support for those suffering from HIV and drug abuse. Drug abuse not only affects the health and well-being of users and their families, but it also affects the health and well-being of our society. In poor urban communities, for example, drugs are responsible for much of the violence and crime and the spread of serious infectious diseases such as AIDS. Although no one is immune to drug addiction, poor and minority populations have been hardest hit by the disease.

Drugs such as marijuana, alcohol, heroin, and cocaine produce mind-altering effects that people may find temporarily satisfying, and they continue to use the drugs as a result. Although many people are at risk of becoming addicted to psychoactive drugs, there is no "addictive personality." Drug addiction, however, has common behavioral features. Younger people are more likely to become addicted to drugs than older people. Additionally, drug addicts usually experience several relapses before they are finally able to break free of the drug's grasp on their minds and bodies.

Characteristics of Addiction

How does one know if he or she is addicted to a drug? A drug addict engages in the inappropriate use of one or more mind-altering drugs repeatedly over time, and this behavior dominates and drives the person's behavior and life. Drug abuse often destroys the addict's relationships, career, health, and life. Despite experiencing these negative effects, the addict continues to engage in the self-destructive behavior. Scientists are just starting to learn why.

Heredity and environment play important roles in determining an individual's risk of drug addiction. People who are described as "thrill seekers" may have a form of a gene that makes their brains respond more positively to dopamine, a neurotransmitter that produces pleasurable sensations. Thus, these individuals are at risk for abusing drugs because the behavior elicits such a positive response. A person, however, is not likely to become addicted to a mind-altering drug unless that substance is readily available in his or her environment.

Escaping the Web

For most people, breaking an addiction is a difficult process. The habitual nature of using the drug, the positively reinforcing sensations, the drug addict's characteristics and environment, and the discomfort of withdrawal make quitting the use of a psychoactive substance difficult to achieve. Through counseling, education, and sometimes the use of medications, many people are able to escape the grip of addiction. Although relapses commonly occur, they are not a sign of failure but an expected aspect of the process of recovery. Most health experts think former addicts must be completely abstinent from all mind-altering drugs if they are to maintain a healthy lifestyle. Since families and friends have been affected by the addiction, they often can play important supportive roles by helping promote drug abstinence.

Assignments

❍ Read Chapter 7, "Drug Use and Abuse," in Alters & Schiff, *Essential Concepts for Healthy Living*, 4th edition. You may find it helpful to take notes on your reading. Then read the Learning Objectives and Overview for this lesson. Review the Key Terms below.

❍ Scan the Video Viewing Questions, and then watch the video program for Lesson 11, "Web of Addiction."

❍ After watching the video, answer the Video Viewing Questions and assess your learning with the Self-Test.

❍ Complete the activities for Chapter 7 in the workbook that accompanies the textbook. Your instructor may use these activities as assignments.

Key Terms

The following terms and those defined in Chapter 7 of the textbook are important to your understanding of this unit.

co-morbid	— The simultaneous occurrence of two or more illnesses.
dopamine	— A chemical that transmits information between neurons.

Video Viewing Questions

1. Drug abuse is a disease. How does drug addiction affect families and society? How can you tell if someone is addicted to a mind-altering substance?

2. Genetic and environmental factors influence one's likelihood of abusing drugs. What personality characteristic places children and adults at risk of drug addiction? How does a person's environment contribute to drug abuse? What role does self-esteem play in substance abuse?

3. Which *illegal* drugs are most likely to be abused, and what are their ill effects?

4. Sandra McDonald states, "Once a person gets into the grip of it...[he or she finds] a comfort level. And anytime you find a comfort level...getting high...is to escape." What does she mean by "getting high is to escape"? Why do addicts continue to abuse drugs, even after their lives have been destroyed by their behavior?

5. Multiple forms of therapy are often needed to help people free themselves from addictive substances. What are these different types of therapies?

6. According to Dr. McCaul, people can recover from a drug addiction by learning new skills. What are these skills? How are *relapses* handled?

Self-Test

Multiple Choice

1. Which of the following inherited characteristics increases a person's risk of drug addiction?
   a. Tall and lean body build
   b. Thrill-seeking personality
   c. Average intelligence
   d. Higher than average metabolic rate

2. Neurotransmitters are necessary for a variety of brain functions including learning new skills and recalling memories. Which neurotransmitter functions in areas of the brain that perceive experiences as pleasurable?
   a. Polypeptide A
   b. Kephalin
   c. Euphoriel
   d. Dopamine

3. Jeremy and Jason are 25-year old identical twins. Jeremy abuses alcohol. Which of the following behaviors is Jason most likely to exhibit?
   a. Homosexuality
   b. Interest in weight lifting
   c. Cigarette smoking
   d. Artistic pursuits

4. Which of the following health conditions is highly associated with drug abuse?
   a. Cystic fibrosis
   b. Parkinson's disease
   c. Type I diabetes
   d. Biological depression

5. Dana is addicted to a stimulant drug that is widely available and legal. His addiction does not affect his relationships or his ability to earn a living. If he stops taking his drug, he gets severe headaches. Dana is addicted to
   a. marijuana.
   b. caffeine.
   c. cocaine.
   d. heroin.

6. Which of the following statements is true?
   a. In the United States, cocaine is the most widely used illegal drug.
   b. The results of studies indicate that marijuana does not have any long-term side effects.
   c. People who inject drugs are at risk of contracting infectious diseases such as hepatitis.
   d. Marijuana is one of the most addictive substances known to man.

7. The physical effects of smoking marijuana are similar to those of
   a. smoking tobacco.
   b. drinking caffeinated beverages.
   c. eating chocolate.
   d. injecting heroin.

8. Maggie smoked marijuana almost every night during her freshman year in college. By the end of her second semester, her grades were so poor that she dropped out of school. According to current research regarding the effects of marijuana, which of the following situations provides the best explanation for why she failed to finish college?
   a. Marijuana is a stimulant that increases the metabolic rate, so Maggie probably couldn't sit still enough in her classes to take good notes.
   b. Marijuana is a narcotic that may make users feel tired, so Maggie may have slept through her classes.
   c. Marijuana may impair memory, so Maggie couldn't remember information from her classes to pass exams.
   d. Marijuana may make users so hungry, Maggie wanted to eat food rather than attend classes.

9. Daniel is a drummer in a jazz band. He's addicted to an illegal drug that makes him feel excited, euphoric, and exceedingly talented when he is taking it. The effects of the drug, however, fade rapidly, leaving Daniel feeling very depressed. Daniel is probably using
   a. cocaine.
   b. nicotine.
   c. heroin.
   d. opioids.

10. Which of the following life threatening conditions have been associated with cocaine use?
    a. Esophageal cancer
    b. Spinal paralysis
    c. Heart attack
    d. Alzheimer's disease

11. At a high school reunion, you see one of your classmates whom you haven't seen in 10 years. He admits to you that he takes methadone at a local hospital out-patient clinic because he was addicted to a drug for 5 years. Your former classmate is in the process of getting over a _____ addiction.
    a. cocaine
    b. heroin
    c. marijuana
    d. nicotine

12. Bob is in a drug treatment program for cocaine addiction. At a friend's house, Bob begins to crave the drug when he sees a couple smoking crack cocaine. Bob asks for the pipe and inhales the smoke. Bob's experience is called
    a. hypowillpower.
    b. relapse.
    c. remission.
    d. failure.

Short Answer

13. Cecily and Alicia are freshmen in college. Cecily loves to hang-glide, climb up and rappel down steep rocky cliffs, and ride her motorcycle without a helmet. Alicia likes to garden, take walks in the park, and read books. Unlike Cecily, she would rather ride in a sports utility vehicle (SUV) than on a motorcycle. Which young woman may have a higher risk of drug addiction? Explain why you chose Cecily or Alicia.

14. Medical experts have determined that there are several risk factors for drug addiction. Discuss environmental and biological factors that influence the likelihood that a person will become addicted to a mind-altering drug.

15. Discuss treatments that are available to help people break their addiction. Use treatment of heroin addiction as an example.

Expanded Analysis

1. Children of alcoholics have a greater risk of becoming alcoholics than children of non-alcoholics. Some people argue that environment plays a major role in the development of alcohol abuse; a child who is exposed to an alcohol-abusing parent is likely to learn the behavior. Scientists, however, have determined that alcoholism is inherited to a large extent. How do scientists use studies of identical twins, who have been adopted by different families, to determine the extent to which alcoholism is inherited?

2. What steps can communities take to reduce the problem of drug addiction? Do you think decriminalizing the use of drugs such as marijuana, cocaine, and heroin is the solution to our country's drug problem?

3. Many drug addiction experts, including Dr. McCaul, think that individuals who have undergone drug treatment programs successfully must abstain from using drugs for the rest of their lives. Some people, however, support the idea that former substance abusers, particularly alcoholics, can learn to control their consumption of the addictive substance. Based on what you have learned from this video and from the textbook, do you think former substance abusers can use psychoactive substances without becoming addicted again?

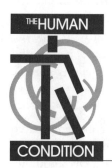

THE **HUMAN**

CONDITION

12

Feels So Good (Hurts So Bad)

Learning Objectives

Upon completing this lesson, you should be familiar with the facts and concepts presented in the lesson and should be able to:

○ Recognize the factors that contribute to a person's susceptibility to alcohol abuse.

○ Describe the effects that alcohol can have on health.

○ Examine at least one major approach that has been successful in treating alcohol abuse.

○ Discuss trends in the use of tobacco products, nationally and internationally.

○ Identify the immediate and long-term health effects of using products that contain tobacco.

○ Compare strategies to help people stop smoking.

Overview

When Americans think of drugs, they usually think of illicit drugs such as cocaine, narcotics, or marijuana. Alcohol and nicotine, however, are legal drugs that cause more health problems for Americans than all illicit drugs combined. In fact, cigarette smoking is the leading cause of preventable death in the United States.

Ten to fifteen percent of people who drink alcohol experience problems as a result. The person who abuses alcohol often uses the drug in dangerous situations, such as when driving or operating other machinery. Additionally, alcohol consumption is often involved in cases of violence and neglect.

Alcohol

People who abuse alcohol are at risk of becoming addicted to the drug. Alcohol addiction (alcoholism) is a complex chronic disease that is difficult to treat. Biological, environmental, and personal factors play important roles in the development of this disease. (Table 8-2 in the textbook lists typical symptoms of alcohol addiction.)

Treating
Alcoholism

Treatment for alcoholism may include hospitalization in a treatment facility, medication, counseling, and self-help groups. An objective of counseling is to teach alcoholics strategies for avoiding the drug. According to Dr. McCaul, alcoholics need to learn "…skills in terms of avoiding people, places, and things that put them at risk." As in the case of other drug addictions, chronic relapses are typical, but people can recover from alcoholism.

Tobacco Use

Of all the mind-altering substances that humans use, the nicotine in tobacco is among the most addictive. Although nicotine produces pleasurable effects in the brain, its effects on the rest of the body are deadly. Over 400,000 Americans die each year as a result of tobacco use. In the United States, tobacco use is responsible for about 30 percent of all cancer deaths each year.

Tobacco use contributes to heart attack, stroke, emphysema, chronic bronchitis, osteoporosis, and gum disease. Despite all the evidence about the harmful effects of tobacco, smoking rates are climbing, especially among American teenagers. According to Dr. Miotto, "The earlier you start smoking, the harder it is to stop smoking."

Since it's difficult to stop using tobacco products, health experts recommend a combination of treatments that may include smoking cessation programs, nicotine patches, and anti-depressants. Smokers who have "kicked the habit" or are in the process of quitting need to anticipate situations that encourage cigarette use and learn strategies and skills that will help them avoid relapses.

Despite their awareness of tobacco's harmful effects on health and despite the difficult process of quitting, many former smokers report that they miss cigarettes. Dr. George Bigelow, Director of the Behavioral Pharmacology Research Unit at Johns Hopkins University School of Medicine, notes, "The memories [and] the learning are always going to be there. The individual is… permanently changed by an experience of addiction." The message is simple: The only way to prevent becoming permanently altered by an addiction is to avoid using the addictive substance.

Assignments

❍ Read Chapter 8, "Alcohol and Tobacco," in Alters & Schiff, *Essential Concepts for Healthy Living*, 4th edition. You may find it helpful to take notes on your reading. Then read the Learning Objectives and Overview for this lesson. Review the Key Terms below.

❍ Scan the Video Viewing Questions, and then watch the video program for Lesson 12, "Feels So Good (Hurts So Bad)."

❍ After watching the video, answer the Video Viewing Questions and assess your learning with the Self-Test.

❍ Complete the activities for Chapter 8 in the workbook that accompanies the textbook. Your instructor may use these activities as assignments.

Key Terms

The following terms and those defined in Chapter 8 are important to your understanding of this unit.

antabuse — A medication that makes people feel nauseous when the drink alcohol.

naltrexone — A medication that reduces an alcoholic's craving for alcohol.

Video Viewing Questions

1. What factors influence a person's vulnerability to alcoholism? Which personality traits are associated with an increased risk of alcoholism?

2. When alcohol is consumed in small amounts, how does it affect the mind and body? How does alcohol withdrawal affect the alcoholic's drinking behavior?

3. Compare the number of drinks consumed per week by "very light" and "light to moderate" drinkers. What is binge drinking behavior?

4. What effects does alcohol consumption have on the body? What are signs of alcohol dependence? What skills does the alcoholic need to develop to recover?

5. What factors contribute to making nicotine so addictive? What effect does using tobacco have on the body? Each year, how many Americans die from smoking-related causes?

6. What are the recommended ways to quit smoking? Why do smokers have such a difficult time quitting the habit?

Self-Test

Multiple Choice

1. According to Dr. Bigelow, children of alcoholic parents have about _____ times the risk of becoming alcoholics, when compared to children of non-alcoholic parents.
   a. 3
   b. 6
   c. 9
   d. 12

2. Which of the following personality traits is associated with increased risk of alcoholism?
   a. Artistic
   b. Intelligent
   c. Hyperactive
   d. Assertive

3. Fernando is uncomfortable in social situations. As soon as he arrives at a party, he heads straight to the bar for an alcoholic drink. Why is Fernando able to socialize and relax after having one drink?
   a. Small amounts of alcohol make people less inhibited.
   b. People who drink alcohol are attracted to other people who drink alcohol.
   c. Alcohol is a stimulant drug that affects the brain stem.
   d. Fernando is better able to control his emotional responses after a drink.

4. At a fraternity party, Jared drank 6 shots of whiskey in two hours. His drinking behavior is classified as
   a. very light.
   b. light.
   c. moderate.
   d. binge.

5. A physician prescribed a medication for Markita that will reduce her craving for alcohol. Markita and her family are hopeful that a combination of the medicine and counseling will help her recover from alcoholism. Which of the following drugs did Markita's physician prescribe?
   a. Phenobarbital
   b. Naltrexone
   c. Inderol
   d. GHB

6. Yesterday, Sam woke up to find himself under some bushes in the back yard of a house. The night before, he attended a Mardi Gras party that was two blocks away from his present location. He can't recall what happened at the party or how he got to the back yard of this stranger's house. Sam's inability to remember what happened is an example of
   a. dementia.
   b. early Alzheimer's disease.
   c. TIA.
   d. blackout.

7. The best-known alcoholism recovery program in the United States is
   a. Alcoholics Anonymous.
   b. Twelve Steps to Freedom.
   c. Recovery Road.
   d. Booze Watchers.

8. According to Dr. Bigelow, people report that _____ use is more addictive than heroin or cocaine use.
   a. marijuana
   b. caffeine
   c. tobacco
   d. alcohol

9. Which of the following statements is true?
   a. The blood-brain barrier prevents nicotine from entering the brain.
   b. Most cases of lung cancer are the result of cigarette smoking.
   c. Each year about 100,000 Americans die of smoking-related illnesses.
   d. Only cocaine, heroin, and alcohol are more addictive than nicotine.

10. The majority of adult smokers started the habit

    a. before they were 18 years of age.

    b. when they were between 18 and 21 years of age.

    c. when they were between 21 and 25 years of age.

    d. after they were 25 years of age.

11. Which off the following statements is true?

    a. Since 1990, smoking rates of American teenagers dropped by 50 percent.

    b. People who started smoking after they were 18 years of age have more difficulty stopping the habit than those who started smoking before they were 18 years old.

    c. Even when smokers quit using tobacco, their risk of heart disease remains very high.

    d. Men who smoke cigarettes have a higher risk of impotence than men who are non-smokers.

12. According to Dr. Bigelow, what are the characteristics of good smoking cessation programs?

    a. A good treatment program combines psychosocial and pharmacological support.

    b. A good treatment program requires smokers to undergo electroshock therapy.

    c. A good treatment program involves hospitalizing the smoker for at least 2 weeks to isolate the addict from other cigarette users.

    d. A good treatment program requires smokers to smoke several packs of cigarettes while sitting in a small, poorly ventilated room every day.

Short Answer

13. Victoria's parents suspect that she could be an alcoholic. Discuss the signs of alcoholism.

14. Discuss the effects that heavy drinking of alcohol can have on the body.

15. Ben is a 49-year-old man who began smoking cigarettes when he was 14 years old. Now he smokes about two packs a day. Describe the effects that smoking cigarettes can have on Ben's body.

Expanded Analysis

1. Compare typical European and American patterns of alcohol consumption. Explain the difference in consumption patterns.

2. According to Dr. Paul McHugh, Director of the Department of Psychiatry and Behavioral Sciences and Psychiatrist-in-Chief at Johns Hopkins University Hospital, people respond differently to drinking small amounts of alcohol. Explain how a person's response to a small amount of alcohol influences his or her vulnerability to alcoholism.

3. Dr. Miotto says, "Addiction is a chronic relapsing disease." Explain what she means.

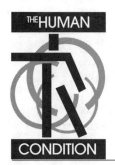

THE HUMAN
CONDITION

13

What You Don't Know...

Learning Objectives

Upon completing this lesson, you should be familiar with the facts, terms, and concepts presented in the lesson and should be able to:

○ Contrast the effects that air pollution and water pollution have on health.

○ Suggest some simple steps that people can take to protect themselves against water-borne pathogens.

○ Give examples of hazardous conditions in the workplace that may endanger the short- and long-term well-being of employees.

○ Discuss the role of government in protecting the environment.

○ Apply at least one strategy to improve the safety of your home environment.

Overview

Pollution is not a problem just in the United States; it is a worldwide problem. The quality of the environment in which people live, work, and play has a major impact on the quality of their lives and health. A polluted environment can result in a variety of health problems. In countries with inadequate water sanitation facilities, water-borne parasites and microbes pose widespread and serious threats to health. In the United States, however, exposure to toxic chemicals is the major environmental health concern. Art Craigmill, a toxicologist at the University of California–Davis, says, "We're exposed to hundreds and thousands of chemicals. So the question is, what happens when we have all of these added together in varying amounts?"

The primary airborne substances that are harmful to humans are sulfur dioxide (SO_2), nitrogen dioxide (NO_2), carbon monoxide (CO), and particulates—small solid particles that are dispersed in the air. Although the ozone (O_3) layer in the upper atmosphere protects people by blocking some of the sun's harmful ultraviolet radiation, breathing ozone is harmful. Industrial and automobile emissions are the major sources of air pollutants, including ozone and carbon monoxide.

Air and Water Pollution

For people with asthma, poor air quality often triggers breathing difficulties. Over time, however, even healthy people suffer the ill effects of air pollution. Long-term exposure to air pollutants contributes to the development of serious lung diseases. According to John Peters, Director of the Division of Occupational and Environmental Medicine at the University of Southern California, breathing particulate matter, nitrogen dioxide, and other nitrogen oxides has more serious long-term effects on health than ozone.

In the United States, sanitation of public drinking water has significantly reduced the risk of water-borne illnesses. In underdeveloped countries, however, the lack of clean drinking water contributes to parasitic infections and diarrheal diseases that sicken or kill many children and adults each year. Learning how these diseases are spread and the use of simple methods of treating water that can reduce the risk of water-borne illnesses would greatly benefit the people living in these countries.

For hundreds of years, people have used oceans as garbage dumps and sewage outflows. This practice continues today as many countries and industries continue to discharge untreated sewage and wastes into seas, polluting nearby beaches and watersheds. Although the sanitation process of public drinking water is regulated in the United States, untreated water from farms, roads, and residential areas eventually enters rivers, lakes, and oceans. Such run-off often contains pesticide residues, animal wastes, and harmful chemicals that seep from storage sites or trash dumps. Swimming or surfing in polluted areas can cause skin rashes and infections, including hepatitis A.

Pollution in the Workplace

Toxic or unsafe workplaces threaten the lives and well-being of workers in many parts of the world. For example, people who work with pesticides and certain solvents, metals, plastics, and adhesives may be poisoned accidentally. Contaminated indoor air and inadequate ventilation are thought to be the causes of sick building syndrome, which includes a host of symptoms reported by occupants of large buildings. In the United States, however, workplaces are much safer than in the past. The federal Occupational Safety and Health Administration (OSHA) protects employees from exposure to health hazards by regulating procedures in business and industry. OSHA employees conduct inspections of businesses that use hazardous materials, and employees of these companies can report violations of proper procedures to OSHA. Many large industries hire industrial hygienists to monitor employee health, identify potentially harmful conditions, recommend actions that correct the hazards, and conduct safety education programs for workers.

Exposure to chronic loud noise can result in hearing loss. (Table 16-3 in the textbook lists common environmental sounds and their intensities.) Although noise pollution is a problem in some environments, measures can be taken to protect against hearing loss. In the machine shops at Boeing, for example, workers must wear special ear protection devices. Outside of the work environment, exposure to sources of intense noise, such as loud music, also can damage hearing. Avoiding excessive noise levels or wearing proper protective devices when exposure is unavoidable can help preserve hearing.

Dangers Lurking in Your Home

We think of our homes as safe havens, but most households contain a supply of improperly stored toxic chemicals. Each year, thousands of young children are poisoned by ingesting common household cleaning compounds, pesticides, lead paint, houseplants, cosmetics, and pharmaceuticals. Dr. Michael Bryant of the Division of Pediatrics at Children's Hospital, Los Angeles, notes "...prevention [is] the key, and looking for...hidden dangers in your home that kids can get into." Taking steps to keep toxic household substances out of the reach of children is the key to prevention.

Even when responsible adults keep hazardous materials away from children, exposure to toxic chemicals can occur. For example, inappropriate use of pesticides to eradicate household pests can result in serious health problems for human residents of a dwelling. Using certified exterminators and carefully follow instructions for the safe use of pesticides can help in the prevention of such incidents.

Increased awareness about the health risks associated with living, working, and playing in polluted environments, encourages people to take steps to reduce exposure to hazardous materials or conditions. By purchasing foods grown without pesticides, for example, consumers can stimulate farmers to produce such crops. In some instances, legislation is necessary to regulate polluters and clean up the environment. The best legacy each generation can leave to the next is a healthy environment.

Assignments

❍ Read Chapter 16, "Environmental Health," in Alters & Schiff, *Essential Concepts for Healthy Living*, 4th edition. You may find it helpful to take notes on your reading. Then read the Learning Objectives and Overview for this lesson. Review the Key Terms below.

❍ Scan the Video Viewing Questions, and then watch the video program for Lesson 13, "What You Don't Know..."

❍ After watching the video, answer the Video Viewing Questions and assess your learning with the Self-Test.

❍ Complete the activities for Chapter 16 in the workbook that accompanies the textbook. Your instructor may use the activities as assignments.

Key Terms

The following terms and those defined in Chapter 16 of the textbook are important to your understanding of this unit.

decibel (dB)	— Unit of measurement for the intensity of sound.
dermal	— Pertaining to the skin.
EPA	— The Environmental Protection Agency.
methyl parathion	— An agricultural pesticide that can be toxic to humans.
NO$_2$	— Nitrogen dioxide, an air pollutant.
NOX	— Nitrogen oxides; compounds that contain nitrogen and oxygen.
OSHA	— The Occupational Safety and Health Administration.
ozone (O$_3$)	— An air pollutant.

phlegm   — Thick mucus secreted by the respiratory tract.

systemic   — Affecting the entire body.

Video Viewing Questions

1. The California Air Resources Board is conducting a study of school-aged children living in Southern California. What is the purpose of this study? Why are children rather than adults being studied?

2. According to Dr. Bennett, how do poor water sanitation systems and the lack of refrigeration affect the health of people in underdeveloped countries? What can these people do to reduce their risk of parasitic infections such as Guinea worm infection?

3. Although ocean water may appear to be clean, contamination with pollutants from human practices and industry is a global problem. What are some of the acute and long-term health problems associated with swimming in polluted water?

4. What can a person do if his or her employer is ignoring health and safety regulations?

5. Why are homes unsafe environments, especially for small children?

6. What happened when the toxic pesticide methyl parathion was used inappropriately in homes to kill roaches? Why does this chemical pose more of a risk to homeowners than to farmers?

7. What can an individual do to rid their homes of pests without harming themselves?

Self-Test

Multiple Choice

1. Which of the following is a major source of air pollution in the United States?
   a. Automobile emissions
   b. Southern pine forests
   c. Pig farming
   d. Synthetic fertilizers

2. Results of the study investigating the effects of air pollution on school-aged children in Southern California indicate that children who live in high air pollution areas
   a. have faster than normal rates of lung growth.
   b. are more likely to be affected by air pollution if they have asthma.
   c. grow taller and weigh less than children living in low air pollution areas.
   d. experience higher rates of attention deficit disorder than children living in low air pollution areas.

3. Benjamin lives in a rural village in Africa. His two young children are among twenty youngsters who have died from diarrheal diseases this year. Each year, several children from his village sicken and die. Which of the following environmental hazards is probably linked to these deaths?

   a. Lead paint chips in the soil where the children played.

   b. Nitrogen dioxide in the air breathed by the children.

   c. Parasitic microoganisms in the water used to wash the children's food.

   d. Viruses spread by monkeys that live in the jungles near the children's homes.

4. According to Donald Hopkins, Associate Executive Director of the Carter Center, what is the best way for villagers to prevent Guinea worm infection?

   a. Eat a high protein, low-fat diet

   b. Get vaccinated

   c. Refrigerate raw foods

   d. Drink bore well water

5. Which of the following statements is true?

   a. Each year, millions of people die as a result of air pollution in under-developed countries.

   b. Ozone pollution is associated with high absenteeism among California school children.

   c. Lack of refrigeration is associated with an increased risk of diarrheal diseases.

   d. Guinea worm infestation is a major public health threat to the water supplies of the United States.

6. You work in a small room with 5 printing presses. While the presses are running, the noise in the room is very loud. You've asked your boss to supply protective ear coverings, but he doesn't seem to be interested in purchasing them for his employees. You're worried about your hearing. Which agency should you contact to report the problem?

   a. OSHA

   b. ONDCP

   c. OFTC

   d. OEEO

7. Your home is infested with termites. Which agency can you contact for information concerning the appropriate pesticide to use?

   a. OAA

   b. FTC

   c. EPA

   d. TOC

8. According to Milton Clark, a toxicologist with the Environmental Protection Agency, which single message would his agency most like people to know and follow concerning pesticide use?

a. When storing pesticides, use brightly labeled containers that children can't open.

b. When choosing pest exterminators, deal with reputable, properly licensed workers.

c. When using pesticides, limit the types used to those that are compatible with your needs.

d. When applying pesticides, don't breathe the material.

Matching

Match the terms with the definitions that follow.

a. methyl parathion
b. lead
c. guinea worm
d. nitrogen dioxide

_____ 9. Air pollutant

_____ 10. Agricultural pesticide

_____ 11. Toxin found in old paint

_____ 12. Parasite

Short Answer

13. A rural village in Southeast Asia has no source of clean water. Villagers drink the same water in which they bathe, swim, and wash their clothes. Each year, many of the villagers die from diarrheal and parasitic infections. What could these people do to make their water safer to drink?

14. An acquaintance of yours offers to spray your house to kill roaches. Discuss the steps you would take to make sure this person does not poison you and your family.

15. You've bought an old house. While moving into it, you notice that the interior of the house has an odd odor, especially in the draperies. Within a few weeks, you develop headaches and nausea; your 10-month old child is fussy and refuses to eat. This child crawls around the house. Her hands and knees have a rash on them. After ruling out infectious agents, your baby's physician suggests an environmental toxin in your house. One of your neighbors tells you that the previous owner complained that the house was infested with carpenter ants. In the basement of the house, you find several mayonnaise jars containing a strong smelling chemical. The draperies have the same odor. You contact the EPA for help. An analysis of the chemical in the jars indicates that it's methyl parathion. You suspect that your house is contaminated with this chemical. Discuss the steps you would have to take to rid your house of this poisonous material.

Expanded Analysis

1. The problem of environmental pollution appears to be overwhelming. What can individuals do to make their environment safer?

2. You buy a home in a "nice" neighborhood; your workplace appears to be clean and safe; your children play in unpolluted areas. Why should you be concerned about pollution?

3. A radio show host interviews a person who claims to be a nutrition expert. This person states that our food supply is polluted as a result of conventional farmers using artificial pesticides, synthetic fertilizers, and growth-stimulating hormones. This person claims that rising cancer rates in the United States provide proof that these compounds are harmful. What do you think of this person's claims?

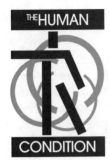

THE HUMAN CONDITION

14

Food for Thought

Learning Objectives

Upon completing this lesson, you should be familiar with the facts, terms, and concepts presented in this lesson and should be able to:

❍ Identify the major classes of nutrients and the roles each plays.

❍ Give examples of foods that are rich sources of complex carbohydrates; of complete proteins.

❍ Name at least three plant foods that provide a good source of protein and can be substituted for animal products rich in protein.

❍ Recognize the importance of vitamins and minerals in the diet, and the conditions that may result when there is an insufficient amount of iron; of calcium.

❍ Identify foods that are rich sources of antioxidants and phytochemicals, including fiber.

❍ Explain how to use the Healthy Eating Pyramid to plan nutritious menus.

Overview

Although Americans have a wide variety of foods from which to choose, they don't always select nutritious diets. We often choose foods on the basis of what we like to eat and can afford and ignore nutritional value. As a result, many Americans are malnourished or marginally nourished, because they eat foods that supply excess energy from fat and barely enough vitamins and minerals.

Nutrients are substances in foods that have important functions in the body. Foods contain six classes of nutrients: carbohydrates, proteins, lipids, vitamins, minerals, and water. Table 9-1 in the textbook provides information concerning the major roles and food sources of the six classes of nutrients.

Plant foods are rich sources of carbohydrates, the body's preferred source of calories (energy). Carbohydrates should supply 50 to 60 percent of daily calories. In addition to carbohydrates, plant foods also provide beneficial non-nutrients such as phytochemicals, including fiber. Table 9-2 in the textbook lists certain phytochemicals and their major food sources; Table 9-4 lists some fiber-rich foods.

The body uses protein to build tissues and to make antibodies, certain hormones, and other compounds. The average person needs about 12 percent of his or her daily calories from protein. According to Ms. Gigliotti, Registered Dietitian and Coordinator of the University of California–Irvine, Weight Management Program, "We will really get enough protein from taking about five to six ounces of meat per day." The typical American diet, however, supplies excessive amounts of protein, especially from animal foods. Instead of relying heavily on animal foods for protein, you can substitute plant sources of this nutrient, such as legumes, nuts, and seeds.

The primary role of fat is to supply energy; many cells burn fatty acids as well as glucose for energy. A healthy diet supplies no more than 30 percent of calories from fats and oils. Diets that contain high amounts of saturated fatty acids are associated with increased risk of heart disease and certain cancers. However, diets that contain high amounts of monounsaturated fatty acids reduce the risk of heart disease. See Table 9-5 for a list of fatty acid contents of commonly eaten fats and oils.

Although vitamins, minerals, and water do not supply calories, these nutrients play other essential roles in the body. Many vitamins and minerals regulate chemical reactions that take place in cells. Vitamins C and E are antioxidants that protect certain cellular material from being damaged by reactive substances such as free radicals. Tables 9-7 and 9-9 provide information about major vitamins and minerals. People often overlook water as an important nutrient. You can live for months without proteins and vitamins but only a few days without water. Water participates in many chemical reactions that take place in cells. In addition to tap water, beverages and most foods are sources of water.

Foods vs. Supplements

Nutritionists use the Recommended Dietary Allowances (RDAs) to evaluate the nutritional adequacy of a population's diet. The average consumer, however, will find it easier to use the Healthy Eating Pyramid—newly revised and updated in 2005 to better reflect current lifestyles—to judge the nutritional quality of his or her diet (see Figure 9-5). Additionally, the consumer can learn specific information about the nutritional content of packaged foods by reading nutrient labels.

Are vitamin and mineral supplements necessary? Many healthy Americans routinely take nutrient supplements in the form of pills or powders in place of foods. Although some people such as pregnant women and vegetarians need to take extra amounts of certain vitamins and minerals, large amounts of these nutrients (megadoses) can be toxic. Registered dietitian Joanne Ikeda notes, "Pills are not a substitute for good nutrition because many of the essential nutrients cannot be isolated, synthesized, and put into a pill."

Scientists are now investigating whether antioxidant nutrients and compounds found in plants (phytochemicals) can prevent or treat a variety of health problems. Antioxidants protect certain cellular compounds from the destructive effects of free radicals and other oxidizing agents. Many phytochemicals act as antioxidants. Presently, scientists are uncertain about the safety of long-term antioxidant use. Nutrition experts recommend eating

4. A person eats a meal containing yogurt, lean meat, soybeans, and eggs. Which of these foods is a rich source of phytochemicals?
   a. Yogurt
   b. Lean meats
   c. Soybeans
   d. Eggs

5. Baked beans, sliced turkey breast, cheddar cheese, and green peas are among the foods offered in a buffet. You want to eat foods that are low-fat sources of protein. Which food is a high-fat source of protein?
   a. Baked beans
   b. Turkey breast
   c. Cheddar cheese
   d. Green peas

6. Which of the following statements is true?
   a. The energy value of a food is reported as a number of BTUs.
   b. Tough chewy meats are good sources of fiber.
   c. Today Americans use the Basic Four Food Groups to plan nutritious menus.
   d. Many Americans suffer from overnutrition, a form of malnutrition.

7. Which of the following foods makes a complete source of protein by combining two *incomplete* protein sources?
   a. Red beans and rice
   b. Cheese and crackers
   c. Steak and potatoes
   d. Beans and ground beef

8. Which of the following statements is true?
   a. If you eat more protein than you need, the extra amino acids are eliminated in urine.
   b. The body uses extra protein to build more muscles.
   c. Cells can burn protein for energy.
   d. The liver converts excess dietary protein into vitamins.

9. Which of the following foods is a good source of fiber?
   a. Margarine
   b. Whole grain bread
   c. Liver
   d. Low-fat milk

Match the terms with the definitions that follow.   **Matching**

    a. antioxidant
    b. fiber
    c. amino acid

____ 10. Chemical unit that makes up proteins

____ 11. Compounds that prevent or reduce the formation free radicals

____ 12. Indigestible plant material

Short Answer

13. According to the Nutrition Facts label, a serving of food contains 180 calories and 15 grams of fat. Each gram of fat provides 9 calories. What percentage of calories in this food are from fat? (Show your calculations.) Explain why you would or would not choose to eat a serving of this food.

14. The following list is a record of everything Joe ate in one day. Analyze Joe's food choices. According to the recommendations of the Healthy Eating Pyramid, did Joe include enough servings of foods from the main food groups? If not, identify foods that he could eat to improve his intake.

( ) 2 cans of sugar-sweetened soda
( ) 2 doughnuts
( ) 1 slice cheese pizza
( ) 4 breadsticks
( ) 1 tablespoon of butter
( ) ¼ cup nacho sauce
( ) 1 chocolate candy bar
( ) 1 bag of corn chips
( ) 8 oz. T-bone steak
( ) 1 baked potato
( ) iced tea
( ) 6 chocolate chip cookies

15. Review the list of foods that Joe ate. What advice would you give Joe to improve his diet?

Expanded Analysis

1. Record what you eat for meals in a typical day. Use Figure 9-5 in the textbook to determine if your intake meets the recommended servings of each of the food groups in the Healthy Eating Pyramid. Did you meet or exceed the recommended number of servings for each of the major food groups? If not, which food groups did not meet the recommended minimum number of servings? What foods could you eat to raise your intake of the "low" food groups?

2. Joanne Ikeda, Nutrition Education Specialist, University of California–Berkeley, states that nutritional advice changes over time. For example, nutritionists no longer recommend that people consume large amounts of polyunsaturated fat. Why do you think nutritionists change their dietary recommendations?

3. Do you complain that you do not "have enough time" to prepare nutritious meals? How can you arrange your time and work environment to help you select a more nutritious diet?

4. Do you eat breakfast? Why is breakfast an important meal?

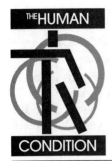

THE HUMAN

CONDITION

15

Weighing In

Learning Objectives

Upon completing this lesson, you should be familiar with the facts and concepts presented in this lesson and should be able to:

○ Identify major health problems associated with excess body fat.

○ Describe methods use to determine if a person is obese.

○ Explain how biological, environmental, social, and psychological factors influence the development of excess body weight.

○ Distinguish between android and gynecoid types of fat distribution and how they affect health.

○ Compare and contrast various weight loss methods, including fad diets.

○ Specify the characteristics of a sound weight loss program.

Overview

An epidemic is spreading across the United States. It's not an infectious disease, but the condition contributes to serious health problems. Poor food choices and sedentary lifestyles have contributed to the dramatic increase in the prevalence of this disease since the 1970s. The disease is obesity. According to Dr. Ralph Cygan, a professor at the University of California–Irvine's College of Medicine, "Today there are more than 100 million Americans who are either overweight or obese...I think we have a very serious public health problem on our hands that we need to address as a nation."

Obesity is a condition characterized by excess body fat. Since it is not easy to directly measure body fat, health experts use the body mass index (BMI) to determine if one is obese. The BMI correlates body size with the risk of developing the chronic conditions that are associated with obesity. Healthy BMIs are in the 19 to 25 range; BMIs of between 25 and 29.9 are in the overweight range. A person with a BMI of 30 or more is obese. Chapter 10 in your text includes a formula for determining BMI. The average American has a BMI of more than 26, which is in the overweight range.

In the United States, the major causes of early morbidity and mortality are strongly associated with obesity. These causes include hypertension; diabetes, and high cholesterol, especially high levels of LDL (low density lipoprotein), the so-called "bad cholesterol." These health conditions are major risk factors for heart disease; the number one killer of Americans.

As one's BMI increases, so does the risk of heart disease. Furthermore, obese people have higher risks of certain cancers and osteoarthritis than non-obese people. Osteoarthritis is a degenerative disease of the joints, especially weight-bearing joints of the lower extremities. It is a major cause of disability among older Americans.

The Battle of the Bulge

Biological, psychological, cultural, and social factors play important roles in the development of obesity. Biological factors, particularly genetics, are involved in the regulation of metabolism and appetite. According to Dean Hamer, Ph.D. and author of *Living with Our Genes*, "...the same genes that control metabolism also control appetite...these genes [code for the production of] hormones and receptors that are released in response to how much a person eats and how fat their cells are...." Thus, people who inherit metabolisms that burn fat slowly may have difficulty controlling their appetite, and become obese as a result.

Genetic factors also influence the distribution of body fat. People who have most of their body fat distributed in the middle of their bodies (android pattern or "apple" shape) are more likely to have the serious health problems associated with obesity than those who have most of their fat distributed below the waist (gynecoid pattern or "pear" shape). People can determine if they have gynecoid or android patterns of fat distribution by measuring their waist and hip circumferences with a tape measure. (See Figure 10-6 in the textbook.)

The prevalence of childhood obesity is increasing in the United States. Poor eating habits and lack of physical activity are largely responsible for this alarming trend. Dr. Barbara Korsch, Professor of Pediatrics at the University of Southern California says, "...if a child is just watching television...[his] metabolism actually goes down. It's a little bit like hibernation." Furthermore, children (and adults) tend to snack on high calorie foods while watching television. Studies indicate that inactive obese children tend to become inactive obese adults.

Prevention vs. Cure

Americans' obsession with "ideal" weight has spawned a multi-billion dollar industry of weight loss products and dietary supplements. Promoters claim these products can melt fat off the body without strenuous exercise or restrictive diets. However, there are no pills that "melt" body fat. The drug ephedra, a powerful stimulant, was banned by the FDA because of dangerous and sometimes fatal side effects such as high blood pressure, arrhythmias (abnormal heart beats), and chest pain.

What about fad diets—do they work? Fad diets typically include severe caloric restriction and nutritionally unbalanced eating plans. Although high protein diets are popular, protein-rich foods are often high in saturated fat and cholesterol, and excess amounts of protein can overwhelm the liver's ability to process it. Additionally, the kidneys must work harder to eliminate some of the breakdown products of protein. For more information concerning various fad diets, refer to Table 10-3 in the textbook.

Although obese people who follow fad diets often lose weight in the short term, they usually fail to keep the weight off permanently because the diets are difficult to maintain. Many overweight people go on and off fad diets. This results in "yo-yo" dieting, the cyclic pattern of weight loss followed by weight gain. Dr. Cygan notes, "The biggest consequence of diets like this is that it perpetuates the yo-yo cycle of dieting...the patients will lose a few pounds... they'll lose some water weight perhaps. But then quickly they'll become very frustrated because there's nothing fundamentally different about their eating behavior [or] their exercise behavior." As a result of not changing his or her lifestyle, the person regains the weight lost, and sometimes gains even more, so that they weigh more than before going on the fad diet.

Is it possible to lose weight and keep it off? Yes—a small percentage of people lose their excess fat and maintain their reduced body weights over time. According to Linda Gigliotti, Registered Dietician and Coordinator of the University of California–Irvine's Weight Management Program, "There's not one strategy that works for everybody in terms of losing weight." However, the most successful weight loss plans include changing eating and exercise patterns for life. Dr. Cygan says, "When patients come to you for weight loss, many have a short-term orientation. They want to go on a program and then resume their prior lifestyle...Obesity, I think, needs to be looked at as a chronic lifelong condition... There are no quick fixes for obesity."

According to the results of research, successful dieters accept responsibility to lose weight, eat a low fat diet, and burn 2,000 to 3,000 calories a week through exercise. Furthermore, they have an environment that supports their weight control efforts. When it comes to losing weight and keeping it off, these factors are the keys to success.

Until scientists have a better understanding of the biological factors that influence body weight and its management, an effective and safe treatment is unlikely. At present, the best treatment for obesity is to avoid becoming obese.

Assignments

❍ Read Chapter 10, "Body Weight and Its Management," in Alters & Schiff, *Essential Concepts for Healthy Living*, 4th edition. You may find it helpful to take notes on your reading. Then read the Learning Objectives and Overview for this lesson. Review the Key Terms below.

❍ Scan the Video Viewing Questions, and then watch the video program for Lesson 15, "Weighing In."

❍ After watching the video, answer the Video Viewing Questions and assess your learning with the Self-Test.

❍ Complete the activities for Chapter 10, in the workbook that accompanies the textbook. Your instructor may use these activities as assignments.

Key Terms

The following terms and those defined in Chapter 10 of the textbook are important to your understanding of this unit.

android	— Pertaining to the male body.
body mass index (BMI)	— A standard that correlates body weight with the risk of developing chronic health conditions associated with obesity. The formula for BMI is: weight (kg) divided by height^2 (m).
epidemic	— An outbreak of an illness or condition that affects many people and spreads rapidly through a region.
fad diets	— Eating plans that are popular for a time, then quickly lose their widespread appeal.
gynecoid	— Pertaining to the female body.
metabolic rate	— The amount of energy the body requires to fuel vital activities during a specified time.
metabolism	— All chemical reactions that take place in the body.
morbidity	— Illness or abnormal condition.
neurotransmitter	— A chemical that participates in the transmission of nerve impulses between nerve cells.
overweight	— A condition in which the body has too much fat. Overweight persons weigh 10 to 19 percent more than desirable.
obesity	— A condition in which the body has unhealthy amounts of body fat. Obese persons weigh 20 percent or more than their desirable weights.
set point	— Pertains to the theory that a person's level of body fat is predetermined. Once body fat reaches this level, internal mechanisms, such as the metabolic rate, maintain this degree of fatness.

Video Viewing Question

1. Height/weight tables are not reliable for determining body fat. What is the BMI? What is the difference between android and gynecoid distribution of body fat? How does the distribution of body fat affect health?

2. Joanne Ikeda, Nutrition Education Specialist at the University of California–Berkeley, says, "…when there were times of famine, there was a survival advantage for those people who deposited fat." Why would the ability to store excess food energy as body fat provide a survival advantage for a human being? Why has this advantage become a disadvantage for modern humans?

3. What aspects of the American lifestyle contribute to the obesity epidemic? How does television watching contribute to the problem of obesity, especially for children?

4. Is there a "magic pill" or "magic bullet" for treating obesity? Why don't fad diets work? According to Linda Gigliotti, which food groups should form the foundation of a weight loss diet and why?

5. Dr. Cygan says, "Many patients come to a weight loss program with extremely unrealistic ideas about what their goal weight should be." What factors influence a person's weight loss goal? How much weight loss is necessary to achieve positive effects on the health risks associated with obesity?

6. The results of studies indicate that people who lose weight and maintain that loss over a long period share certain characteristics. Which personal characteristics seem to be necessary for one to lose weight and keep it off? What is a "toxic" environment?

Self-Test

Multiple Choice

1. Which of the following individuals is obese?
   a. A man whose BMI is 29
   b. A woman whose BMI is 24
   c. A person with a BMI of 27
   d. A person with a BMI of 30

2. Which of the following conditions is associated with excess body fat?
   a. Diabetes
   b. Multiple sclerosis
   c. Cystic fibrosis
   d. Osteoporosis

3. Which of the following tools is the most reliable to use for estimating one's percentage of body fat?
   a. Bathroom scale
   b. Bioelectrical impedance device
   c. Cloth tape measure
   d. Height-weight table

4. Ben is overweight and has most of his excess fat in the area of his waistline. He jokes about his "spare tire." What would you tell Ben?
   a. He has an android distribution of fat, which is healthier than a gynecoid distribution.
   b. His distribution of fat increases his risk of diverticulosis.
   c. He has a gynecoid distribution of fat, which increases his risk of hypertension.
   d. His distribution of fat increases his risk of diabetes.

5. Which of the following statements about fad diets is true?
   a. People who follow fad diets usually achieve permanent weight loss.
   b. People who follow fad diets typically eat a wide variety of nutritious foods while on the diets.
   c. People who follow fad diets often experience yo-yo cycling of weight loss and gain.
   d. People don't lose weight while following fad diets.

6. One of your friends wants to lose 15 pounds and keep the weight off. This person asks you for advice. After having read Chapter 10 and watching "Weighing In," what is the most sensible advice you can give your friend?
   a. Eat a variety of foods, but make fruits and vegetables the foundation of your diet.
   b. Find a good surgeon and have a gastric bypass operation.
   c. Consume about 400 calories a day on a carbohydrate-free, liquid protein fast.
   d. Take diet pills, jog 3 miles a day, and follow the cabbage soup diet.

7. According to Dr. Cygan, which of the following statements is true?
   a. By losing only 10 percent of their weight, obese people can improve their health.
   b. When caloric intake is very low, the body's metabolic rate increases and fat is burned at a higher rate than normal.
   c. When supervised by physicians, yo-yo dieting results in permanent weight loss.
   d. When protein is injected into obese people, fat melts off their bodies during sleep.

8. When caloric intake is very low, the body
   a. gains lean muscle mass.
   b. stores cellulite around the waistline.
   c. increases its metabolic rate.
   d. burns lean tissues for energy.

9. Which of the following statements is true?
   a. The same genes that control metabolism also control appetite.
   b. Obese people are more likely to suffer from osteoporosis than osteoarthritis.
   c. It is healthier to have an android pattern than a gynecoid pattern of fat distribution.
   d. While watching television, a child's metabolism increases.

Matching

Match the terms with the definitions that follow.
   a. serotonin
   b. body mass index
   c. metabolic rate

_____ 10. A neurotransmitter that affects appetite

_____ 11. The amount of energy the body uses for vital activities during a specified time

_____ 12. Ratio of weight to height

Short Answer

13. What is meant by "apple" shapes and "pear" shapes. Explain how the distribution of body fat affects health.

14. Explain why most people who lose weight regain some or all of the weight within a few years.

15. Bill is thinking about trying the weight loss plan that is promoted in a best-selling diet book. He wants you to help him analyze the plan. Discuss what kinds of information you would need to know about the weight loss plan so you can give him good advice.

Expanded Analysis

1. Have you or someone you know tried to lose weight by following a fad diet? Which fad diets were tried? Were the weight loss efforts successful?

2. "Fat people could lose weight if they would just stop eating." After watching "Weighing In" and reading Chapter 10, what have you learned about obesity and weight control that might cause you to react differently to this statement now?

3. Years ago, people often thought that being overweight was a sign of health and having enough income to eat "rich" foods. A fat baby was a healthy baby. How has our attitudes toward excess body fat changed and why?

4. Since diets to lose weight don't seem to work in the long run, do you think there is too much emphasis on dieting in the United States and not enough emphasis on physical activity? What could be done to inspire Americans to become more physically active?

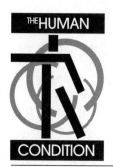

THE HUMAN
CONDITION

16

Working It Out

Learning Objectives

Upon completing this lesson, you should be familiar with the facts, terms, and concepts presented in this lesson and should be able to:

○ Discuss the health benefits of a physically active lifestyle.

○ Identify the major components of health-related physical fitness.

○ Explain the concept of aerobic exercise and name at least five different types of aerobic exercises.

○ Design a personal workout session that includes stretching, warm-up, and cool-down activities.

○ Develop a physical fitness plan that can be followed for a lifetime.

Overview

Orthopedic surgeon Thomas Mirich states, "It has been shown that people who participate in a regular exercise program...have better health overall [than people who do not exercise]." Indeed, the results of numerous studies indicate that people can live longer, healthier lives by increasing their level of physical activity, especially aerobic exercise. A physically active lifestyle reduces the risk of premature death from heart disease, diabetes, hypertension, and certain cancers. Furthermore, physical activity can help prevent obesity, strengthen bones, and improve mood and sense of well-being. Nearly everyone, even elderly people, can derive some health benefits from being more physically active. Most Americans, however, lead sedentary lives.

The health-related components of physical fitness are cardiorespiratory (sometimes called aerobic) fitness, muscular strength, muscular endurance, flexibility, and body composition. Many fitness experts consider cardiorespiratory fitness to be the most important health-related element of physical fitness. Regular aerobic exercise enhances cardiorespiratory fitness, increasing the stroke volume of the heart and reducing the resting heart rate.

Physical Fitness and Health

The need to develop flexibility is often overlooked by people who exercise. Flexible muscles allow joints to move within their normal range of motion. Physical therapist Gregg Olsen says, "If you're not actively doing something to maintain or improve your flexibility, then you're probably going to be tightening up." When done properly, stretching exercises improve flexibility, which increases one's quality of life. Before performing static stretches, one should warm up with light exercise, then stretch gently.

Strong muscles are necessary to achieve good health and well-being but also to be able to participate in most sports. To develop muscular strength, muscles need to be overloaded by repeatedly moving objects that become progressively heavier. Weight training not only increases muscular strength, but also improves peoples' speed, agility, and balance, which are elements of sports-related fitness. Even if you do not participate in sports, weight training can lower your risk for injury when performing routine physical activities, such as carrying small children or heavy grocery bags.

Aerobic activities are important if one is to achieve a high degree of cardiorespiratory fitness. Aerobic activities strengthen the heart, which is a muscle. How can you tell if an activity is aerobic? Aerobic activities involve moving all four limbs together, such as in walking, jogging, and swimming.

When planning an effective overall fitness regimen, people need to consider their goals before choosing exercise activities. For example, weight lifting programs can be tailored to achieve muscle tone if one is not interested in developing muscular bulk. Additionally, individuals should design personal fitness programs that provide health benefits, are enjoyable, satisfy their needs and interests, and can be followed for a lifetime.

Too Much of a Good Thing

Frequently, people begin their fitness program with unrealistic goals. They may try to rush the process of becoming fit and suffer injuries as a result. To reduce the risk of an exercise-induced health problem or injury, unfit middle-aged people should have a physical exam before embarking on a fitness program. After receiving their health care practitioner's approval, people can ask a physical therapist or personal trainer to recommend an appropriate training regimen.

Even seasoned athletes can suffer overuse injuries, particularly of the shoulders and knees. Some injuries can recover with rest, but others require surgery or therapy. Arthroscopic surgeries enable physicians to treat such injuries without making large incisions. Including warm up, stretching, and cool down activities in one's exercise regimen may reduce the risk of injury.

Little Busy Bodies

The typical child seems to be on the move from morning until night. Today's parents, however, often discourage their children from playing outdoors because of safety concerns. By enrolling their children in organized athletic activities such as teams sports, dance, or gymnastics, many parents maintain more control over their childrens' physical activity. Participation in such activities can build childrens' social and physical skills as well as their enthusiasm for being active, but their bodies are not mature enough to handle the physical demands of some activities. As a result, injuries to youngsters' ligaments, tendons, joints, and growth plates at the ends of their bones can occur. Furthermore, parents and coaches who place too much emphasis on excelling may ruin a child's enjoyment of the activity. The goal for parents and adults is to encourage children to enjoy exercise and make it a daily habit.

Throughout life, the body undergoes physical changes. As a result, exercise programs and physical activities may need to change as one ages. Even elderly people, however, can benefit from appropriate exercises. Such activities can help regulate blood sugar, reduce high blood pressure, relieve arthritic stiffness and discomfort, and enhance cardiovascular fitness. A person is never too old to be moving his or her body. To remain healthy, everyone needs to be committed to a physically active lifestyle.

Assignments

○ Read Chapter 11, "Physical Fitness," in Alters & Schiff, *Essential Concepts for Healthy Living*, 4th edition. You may find it helpful to take notes on your reading. Then read the Learning Objectives and Overview for this lesson. Review the Key Terms below.

○ Scan the Video Viewing Questions, and then watch the video program for Lesson 16, "Working It Out."

○ After watching the video, answer the Video Viewing Questions and assess your learning with the Self-Test.

○ Complete the activities for Chapter 11 in the workbook that accompanies the textbook. Your instructor may use these activities as assignments.

Key Terms

The following terms and those defined in Chapter 11 of the textbook are important to your understanding of this unit.

anterior cruciate ligament	— A ligament within the knee joint that stabilizes the joint, preventing the joint from twisting.
arthroscopy	— A form of surgery that repairs injured joints. Surgeons use small incisions and a tiny scope to observe the damage inside a joint and repair it.
ballistic stretching	— Extending a muscle by making jerking or bouncing motions.
proprioception	— The sense of being aware of the body's position.
static stretching	— Extending a muscle by making slow smooth movements.

Video Viewing Questions

1. According to Dr. Mirich, what are the health benefits of regular exercise?

2. Health experts recommend aerobic exercise for cardiorespiratory fitness. How do you distinguish aerobic from non-aerobic activities?

3. What are the health components of fitness? Which health component is often neglected?

4. Weight lifting builds muscular strength and endurance. How do one's goals influence the type of weight lifting regimen one chooses to perform?

5. What kinds of injuries often occur to athletes? To non-athletes? How are these injuries treated?

Self-Test

Multiple Choice

1. The results of numerous studies indicate that regular exercise improves health. People who exercise regularly have a lower risk of
   a. premature death.
   b. fractured ankles.
   c. hepatitis A.
   d. mental illness.

2. According to Dr. Mirich, a regular exercise program improves the functioning of various body organs and tissues. Which of the following conditions may be prevented or improved by exercise?
   a. Anemia
   b. Septicemia
   c. Osteoporosis
   d. Presbyopia

3. Elderly people who exercise regularly have better _____ than elderly people who are sedentary.
   a. Vision
   b. Hearing
   c. Intonation
   d. Balance

4. Research indicates that exercise definitely reduces the risk of ____ cancer.
   a. liver
   b. colon
   c. bladder
   d. brain

5. Sam's physician tells him to perform aerobic exercises. Sam is not sure which exercises are aerobic. Which of the following physical activities would you recommend for Sam?
   a. Yoga
   b. Stretching muscles
   c. Lap swimming
   d. Lifting weights

6. Jamie likes to jog 3 miles every other day. As soon as she leaves her house, she starts jogging at her usual pace. Which health component of fitness has she ignored?
   a. Cardiorespiratory fitness
   b. Flexibility
   c. Speed
   d. Balance

7. According to physical therapist Greg Olsen, which of the following statements is true?
   a. Holding a stretch for 5 seconds is adequate for most adults.
   b. People should warm up by stretching until they feel moderate pain, then hold the stretch for 1 minute, enduring the discomfort.
   c. Stretching will improve flexibility if one is too tight.
   d. Most healthy people do not have to include stretching in their fitness program.

8. Which of the following groups of people should obtain a physician's OK before beginning an exercise regimen?
   a. preschool children
   b. adolescents
   c. young adults
   d. middle-aged adults

Match the terms with the definitions that follow.   **Matching**

   a. static stretching
   b. ballistic stretching
   c. arthroscopy
   d. aerobic

_____   9. A type of surgery that repairs injured joints

_____   10. Stretching by making rapid bouncing motions

_____   11. Oxygen-requiring

_____   12. Stretching by extending the muscle and joint smoothly

13. Explain why exercising for more than an hour can be harmful.   **Short Answer**

14. Judy wants to increase her fitness level. Discuss what she should consider before designing an individualized exercise program.

15. Marie and Mike have a 5-year old daughter, Mandy. They are concerned that Mandy is spending too much time sitting at her computer. Marie would like Mandy to study ballet; Mike played soccer in college and would like his daughter to get involved in the sport so she can get a scholarship to college in 13 years. Discuss what you would tell Marie and Mike about the pros and cons of children becoming intensively involved in athletic endeavors.

Expanded Analysis

1. Does your lifestyle affect your ability to engage in physical activity regularly? Discuss lifestyle modifications that you can make to increase your physical activity level.

2. If the health benefits of exercising do not increase after one hour, why do some people exercise for longer periods?

3. What could be done to encourage owners of large businesses and corporations to establish workplace exercise facilities and programs that would improve the fitness levels of employees? What benefits could employers derive from such facilities and programs?

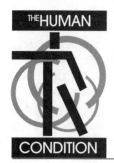

17

Germ Warfare

Learning Objectives

Upon completing this lesson, you should be familiar with the facts and concepts presented in the lesson and should be able to:

○ Discuss the public health role of the Centers for Disease Control and Prevention, and how it has changed through the years.

○ Identify infectious diseases that continue to be serious problems, especially in developing countries.

○ Formulate arguments that support world-wide efforts to eradicate diseases like measles and polio, and recognize the unintended danger such efforts could create.

○ Describe in general terms how public health organizations respond when there is an outbreak of an unidentified disease, and the steps they're taking to recognize isolated outbreaks sooner.

○ List three ways to reduce the risk of contracting infectious diseases.

Overview

Throughout the world, disease control and prevention are major concerns of public health officials. During the last half of the twentieth century, the advent of vaccines and antibiotics reduced the risk of several deadly infectious diseases. As the threat of infectious disease epidemics subsided, scientists at the Centers for Disease Control and Prevention (CDC) in Atlanta, Georgia, turned their attention toward preventing chronic diseases and injuries. The threat of infections, however, has returned. Now, public health officials are fighting a different group of microbes, and this global war against invisible but formidable enemies seems to have no end.

A major challenge facing public health officials is the waning effectiveness of many antibiotics. In the past, antibiotics were extremely useful in killing dangerous bacteria. Over time, however, people misused antibiotics. As a result, some bacteria mutated and became resistant to the deadly effects of antibiot-

The Perpetual Battle

ics. So scientists must continually strive to develop new antibiotics that can kill resistant bacteria. In a sense, scientists are involved in an "arms race" against the microbes.

Vaccines are another important way of combating infectious diseases. Vaccines have eradicated smallpox so that it is no longer a threat. Polio, measles, and tuberculosis are under control in developed nations due to vaccination programs, but these infections still disable and kill many people in developing countries, especially in Africa and Asia. AIDS now kills more people in Africa than any other infectious disease. Medical researchers are trying to develop an effective vaccine that will prevent this terrible disease.

Although scientists may find ways to prevent or cure infectious diseases that have been present for hundreds of years, they also must contend with new or formerly unreported pathogens, such as the hanta virus and *E. coli*. Such pathogens have become worldwide threats as humans travel easily and quickly from distant places, carrying their pathogen load with them.

Containing the Enemy

People can take several steps to reduce the spread of infectious diseases. For example, people can reduce their chances of contracting an infectious disease by being immunized properly, following instructions when using antibiotics, carefully preparing foods that may harbor dangerous microbes, and using insect repellents when outdoors. It may not be possible to eradicate every pathogen, but taking these steps can help reduce your risk of infection.

Assignments

○ Read Chapter 14, "Infection, Immunity, and Noninfectious Disease," in Alters & Schiff, *Essential Concepts for Healthy Living*, 4th edition. You may find it helpful to take notes on your reading. Then read the Learning Objectives and Overview for this lesson. Review the Key Terms below.

○ Scan the Video Viewing Questions, and then watch the video program for Lesson 17, "Germ Warfare."

○ After watching the video, answer the Video Viewing Questions and assess your learning with the Self-Test.

○ Complete the activities for Chapter 14 in the workbook that accompanies the textbook. Your instructor may use these activities as assignments.

Key Terms

The following terms and those defined in Chapter 14 are important to your understanding of this unit.

bio-terrorism	— The deliberate use of infectious agents to kill large numbers of people; "germ warfare."
pathogen	— Infectious disease agents such as viruses and bacteria.
resistance	— Pertaining to a microbe's ability to avoid the deadly effects of an antibiotic.

virulence — Pertaining to the microbes' ease of causing an infection.

Video Viewing Questions

1. What are the public health roles of the Centers for Disease Control and Prevention?

2. What are the most serious infectious diseases in Africa, Asia, and other parts of the world?

3. Antibiotics used to be "silver bullets" in the war against disease-causing bacteria. What happened to reduce the effectiveness of many antibiotics?

4. When describing the outbreak of a virulent strain of *E. coli* 157 bacteria, Dr. Ostroff says, "One of the things that we know with many of the emerging infectious diseases...is that we can tell retrospectively that they're not really new. They're just newly recognized." What does he mean?

5. What is the public health value of the "unexplained death project"? Should Americans be concerned about infectious diseases that originate in foreign countries?

6. What steps can Americans take to reduce their risk of infectious diseases?

Self-Test

Multiple Choice

1. Which federal agency is responsible for monitoring the health status of Americans and tracking infectious diseases in the United States?
   a. The Centers for Disease Control and Prevention
   b. National Institutes of Health
   c. The U.S. Department of Health
   d. The Infectious Disease Control Bureau

2. By the middle of the twentieth century, _____ was no longer a public health threat to people living in the southeastern United States.
   a. AIDS
   b. cow pox
   c. gonorrhea
   d. malaria

3. Which of the following statements is true?
   a. Malaria is still a major public health threat in the United States.
   b. No new case of smallpox has been reported in the world since the 1970s.
   c. In 1995, an agreement between Russia and the United States resulted in destruction of all supplies of the smallpox virus.
   d. Farmers in the Midwestern United States need to be concerned about the threat of the Ebola virus.

4. At one time, malaria was the major cause of death in Africa. Today, _____ is the leading cause of death on the African continent.
   a. AIDS
   b. heart disease
   c. liver cancer
   d. tuberculosis

5. Which infectious disease is the most common cause of death and disability in the world?
   a. AIDS
   b. Heart disease
   c. Tuberculosis
   d. Liver cancer

6. A team of Russian scientists report that a small vial containing smallpox virus is missing from a guarded research facility. American and Russian officials are afraid that the person who stole the vial will release the virus in an elementary school in a Western country. If this person carries out the plan to release the virus, it would be an example of
   a. bio-terrorism.
   b. medical tyranny.
   c. viral weaponry.
   d. pathogenic offensive.

7. Worldwide health organizations often work together to eradicate infectious diseases through immunization programs. Medical experts plan to target _____ after they eliminate the threat of polio.
   a. AIDS
   b. mumps
   c. measles
   d. syphilis

8. Several hours after the Hernandez family reunion picnic ended, Juan Hernandez and his 4-year old cousin Alberto developed severe bloody diarrhea and had to be hospitalized. Alberto almost died. After studying samples of the food served at the picnic, public health officials identified *E. coli* as the source of the infection. Which of the following foods eaten by Juan and Alberto was the most likely source of this deadly bacteria?
   a. Canned, sugar-free soft drink
   b. Double-layered chocolate cake
   c. Partially-cooked hamburger
   d. Canned green beans

9. When planting vegetables, a farmer in a small Korean village uses cow manure as fertilizer. Eventually, the vegetables are imported into the United States. Since you don't like cooked vegetables, you use the fresh Korean vegetables in a salad, without washing them first. These vegetables are probably contaminated with
   a. measles virus.
   b. *E. coli* bacteria.
   c. polio virus.
   d. bacteria that cause pneumonia.

10. A physician gave Jake a 14-day prescription for a sore throat. Jake took the medication for 5 days but discontinued it when his throat felt better. A week later, Jake's sore throat returned. The bacteria that caused the sore throat probably developed
   a. resistance.
   b. endurance.
   c. persistence.
   d. obsolescence.

11. What steps should people take to preserve the effectiveness of antibiotics? **Short Answer**

12. Discuss at least three steps you can take to avoid infectious diseases.

Expanded Analysis

1. In the last half of the twentieth century, physicians widely prescribed antibiotics to treat various infections in the United States. By the beginning of this century, many antibiotics had lost their effectiveness. Explain why.

2. Should the public be concerned about the threat of bio-terrorism? What steps can be taken to reduce this threat?

3. Serious infectious diseases that used to be confined to Africa and Asia are now causing infections in the United States. What factors contribute to the "lack of borders" for infectious disease agents?

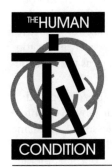

18

The Modern Plague

Learning Objectives

Upon completing this lesson, you should be familiar with the facts and concepts presented in the lesson and should be able to:

○ Recount the emergence of HIV/AIDS in the early 1980s in the United States, and initial efforts to identify a case definition for the disease and its mode of transmission.

○ Explain how HIV affects the body, and what makes it a particularly difficult virus to contain.

○ Identify specific groups of people who are at high risk for contracting HIV, and why.

○ Recognize how treatment modalities for HIV have changed, and explain why its now approaching chronic disease status.

○ Identify ways to reduce your personal risk of contracting HIV.

Overview

In 1981, physicians began to report cases of a mysterious illness that seemed to affect only gay young men. The men were dying from rare cancers and opportunistic infections that did not occur in people with normal immune systems. Alarmed, medical researchers called the deadly disease acquired immunodeficiency syndrome (AIDS) when they determined that the infectious agent disarmed the immune system, rendering it useless.

Within a few years, scientists had identified the human immunodeficiency virus (HIV) as the cause of the disease. The primary methods of HIV transmission were also identified as being through intimate sexual contact, IV drug use, blood transfusion, and placental transfer. One does not become infected with the virus through casual physical contact, blood donation, or insect bites. Scientists also learned that HIV can live for years inside certain immune system cells without causing symptoms of AIDS. Unaware that they are infected, people can transmit the deadly HIV virus to others.

Before the advent of anti-viral medications, a person with AIDS could expect to live only about one to two years. Today, there is no drug that kills HIV, but combinations of medications enable people who are infected with the virus to live fairly normal lives. Medical researchers, however, must continually search for new drugs and approaches to combat HIV, as the virus becomes resistant to current therapies.

In the United States, the number of deaths from AIDS has dropped dramatically over the past few years. Nevertheless, the rate of new HIV infections continues to rise rapidly. Dr. Alexandra Levine, Professor of Medicine at the University of Southern California, is very concerned about the rise of HIV infection among women. She notes, "At the beginning of the epidemic, it was almost unheard of for a woman to have this disease. At this point...[about] 25 percent...of patients with AIDS are women. And women are the fastest rising new group of HIV/AIDS in the country, and probably in the world as well."

Slowing the Epidemic

AIDS is a global epidemic. According to Dr. Ronald Mitsuyasu, Director of the Center for AIDS Research and Education (CARE) at the University of California–Los Angeles, "[AIDS is] decimating populations in parts of Central Africa, in parts of Southeast Asia, in parts of the Indian subcontinent." In these parts of the world, there are not enough resources to reduce the spread of HIV and fight AIDS.

Are medical researchers close to developing a vaccine that will prevent HIV infection? According to Dr. Harold Varmus, former director of the National Institutes of Health, "I do think it will be a long time before we have an adequate vaccine [against HIV]." Given this sobering forecast, many people need to change their attitudes about HIV/AIDS. For example, they need to recognize that AIDS is not a "gay disease;" anyone can contract HIV if they engage in risky behaviors or have sex with people who do. (Table 14-1 in your textbook lists characteristics of high-risk sex partners.) The primary ways people can reduce their risk of contracting the virus is to avoid casual sexual encounters, always use condoms during sexual intercourse, and avoid using illegal IV drugs.

Every American should be concerned about the threat of HIV/AIDS. Until medical researchers develop an effective HIV vaccine or a cure for AIDS, this plague will continue to take millions of lives in the United States and other nations.

Assignments

❍ Review the "Human Immunodeficiency Virus" section of Chapter 14, pages 398–403, in Alters & Schiff, *Essential Concepts for Healthy Living*, 4th edition. You may find it helpful to take notes on your reading. Then read the Learning Objectives and Overview for this lesson. Review the Key Terms below.

❍ Scan the Video Viewing Questions, and then watch the video program for Lesson 18, "Modern Plague."

❍ After watching the video, answer the Video Viewing Questions and assess your learning with the Self-Test.

○ Complete the activities for Chapter 14 in the workbook that accompanies the textbook. Your instructor may use these activities as assignments.

Key Terms

The following terms and those defined in Chapter 14 are important to your understanding of this unit.

IV	— Abbreviation for intravenous; pertaining to injecting drugs into veins.
monogamous	— Having one spouse or sexual partner for a long period of time.
opportunistic infections—	Infectious diseases that people contract when their immune systems have been weakened by other diseases or conditions.

Video Viewing Questions

1. In the early 1980s, physicians in the United States became alarmed at what appeared to be the outbreak of a new disease. How did medical researchers construct a case definition for the disease? Which diseases or conditions define AIDS?

2. After defining AIDS, scientists were able to determine how the virus that causes AIDS spreads. How is HIV transmitted? What are ways that the virus is not transmitted?

3. In the United States, which populations have a high risk of contracting HIV?

4. Although rates of HIV infection are still climbing in the United States, the number of people dying from AIDS is declining. The disease, however, is decimating the populations of some less-developed countries. Why are more people dying of AIDS in less developed countries than in the United States?

5. Medical researchers have identified HIV as the cause of AIDS. Today, people infected with HIV can take a variety of medications to keep its deadly effects at bay, yet the virus remains in their bodies. What makes HIV so deadly? Why have scientists been unable to develop a vaccine that prevents HIV infection or a drug that kills the virus?

6. What can people do to reduce their risk of HIV infection?

Self-Test

Multiple Choice

1. Which of the following statements concerning HIV infection is true?
   a. AIDS is primarily a disease that affects homosexual males.
   b. People with AIDS suffer from rare cancers and opportunistic infections.
   c. In tropical parts of the world, mosquitoes spread HIV.
   d. People can contract HIV by donating blood.

2. After HIV enters the body, it attaches to and infects
   a. red blood cells.
   b. liver cells.
   c. T4 cells.
   d. bladder cells.

3. Three years ago Clayton was infected with HIV. Eventually he'll develop severe infections as a result of his weakened _____ system.
   a. circulatory
   b. digestive
   c. excretory
   d. immune

4. Which of the following groups of Americans comprises the fastest rising new group of HIV-infected persons?
   a. Elderly people
   b. Infants
   c. Homosexuals
   d. Women

5. Indira is infected with HIV; she has just given birth to a baby. Indira is most likely to transmit HIV to her infant when she
   a. changes her baby's diapers.
   b. breast-feeds her baby.
   c. kisses her baby.
   d. bathes her baby.

6. AIDS is a worldwide public health crisis. The disease has decimated populations in certain parts of the world. In which of the following regions or countries is AIDS a major cause of death?
   a. northern Europe
   b. Canada
   c. central Africa
   d. Japan

7. Until recently, _____ was largely responsible for the rapid spread of HIV infections in Thailand.
   a. prostitution
   b. contaminated water
   c. air pollution
   d. alcoholism

8. Which of the following statements is true?
    a. In Thailand, government officials were able to reduce the spread of HIV by opening centers where narcotic addicts could get clean IV needles.
    b. If anti-HIV medications are not taken on schedule, they can become ineffective.
    c. Before he died, Dr. Jonas Salk discovered an effective and safe vaccine that prevents HIV infection.
    d. Dr. Harold Varmus, former director of the National Institutes of Health, predicts that a vaccine against the virus that causes AIDS will be developed soon.

9. According to Dr. Levine, the number one way to protect yourself against HIV is to
    a. use clean needles when you inject IV drugs into your body.
    b. wash your genitals with soap and warm water after sex.
    c. make sure that you get vaccinated against HIV.
    d. know your sexual partner.

10. Discuss how HIV can enter the human body.   **Short Answer**

11. In 1993, Arthur was not aware that he had been infected with HIV. For several years, he felt fine and showed no signs of AIDS. Eventually, he became very ill with opportunistic infections and was diagnosed with AIDS. Explain why HIV infection did not make Arthur ill or cause his death when he was infected years earlier.

12. Explain why many Americans do not think they are at risk for HIV/AIDS.

Expanded Analysis

1. Discuss public health efforts that could slow the spread of HIV in the United States and the rest of the world.

2. Why is there no risk of contracting HIV by donating blood?

3. Explain why it will take a long time to develop an effective vaccine that can prevent HIV infection.

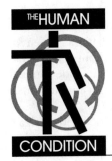

19

Heart of the Matter

Learning Objectives

Upon completing this lesson, you should be familiar with the facts, terms, and concepts presented in the lesson and should be able to:

○ Differentiate between HDL and LDL and the significance of these measurements in relation to coronary artery disease (also referred to as coronary heart disease).

○ Recognize methods of detecting and countering damage caused by atherosclerosis.

○ Describe the signs and symptoms of a heart attack, and how these symptoms may differ for men and women.

○ Identify treatment regimens for people recovering from by-pass surgery or heart attacks.

Overview

Atherosclerosis—hardening and narrowing of the arteries—is the number one cause of death in the United States. Cholesterol-filled plaques in the walls of arteries interfere with normal blood flow by narrowing the passageway through which blood flows and making clots more likely to form. If a clot lodges in a narrowed coronary artery, it causes ischemia. When this happens, the heart muscle supplied by that artery does not receive sufficient oxygen, and the person experiences angina (chest pain). If the flow of blood in a coronary artery is blocked completely, the person has a myocardial infarction, a heart attack.

Table 12-2 in the textbook lists major risk factors for atherosclerosis, including cigarette smoking, diabetes mellitus, physical inactivity, total blood cholesterol levels above 200 mg/dl, low levels of HDL cholesterol, and high levels of LDL cholesterol. Table 12-3 indicates healthy levels of HDL and LDL.

Atherosclerosis: Detecting and Treating the Damage

Physicians have several methods of diagnosing atherosclerosis. An electrocardiogram (EKG) provides a graphic record of the electrical activity of the heart. Stress testing involves the use of EKGs to assess the functioning of the heart during treadmill exercise. If stress testing indicates that the patient's heart is not getting enough oxygen during an intense workout, physicians usually follow up with an angiogram. Other diagnostic tests include cardiac MRI and electron beam CT scan of the heart, which detects calcium deposits, a sign of plaque build-up.

When a few arteries are blocked, surgeons often use balloon catheterization to open the arteries and stents to keep them from narrowing again. Atherectomy or laser devices can remove small pieces of plaque from carotid arteries. Surgeons often perform coronary bypass procedures in patients who have severely blocked coronary arteries.

Heart Attack

Many people with atherosclerosis are unaware of the extent to which their coronary arteries are blocked. When these people have a heart attack, they often deny or ignore their signs and symptoms. The Managing Your Health box in Chapter 12 lists the signs and symptoms of heart attack. In about one out of three heart attack cases, death is the first manifestation of heart disease. Thus, if you or someone you know has signs and symptoms of a heart attack, call 911 or have someone take you or the affected person to a hospital. Dr. Faxon, Chief of Cardiology at the University of Southern California School of Medicine notes that women typically have different signs and symptoms of heart attack than men. Women often complain of indigestion, dizziness and weakness; unlike men, they may have little or no chest pain.

Preventing Atherosclerosis

Dr. Faxon states that, "…if you have heart disease in your family, you need to be more vigilant about making sure that the modifiable risk factors are taken care of. And those are high cholesterol, high blood pressure, cigarette smoking, [and] physical inactivity…" For example, people can often reduce their high LDL cholesterol levels by eating fewer fatty foods, losing weight, and exercising. Table 12-4 lists these and other measures you can take to modify your risk of atherosclerosis.

Risk factors are cumulative; the more that apply to your lifestyle, the greater your chances of having atherosclerosis. Dr. Faxon says "atherosclerosis is a disease of our entire life. And therefore, prevention needs to start early in life, not late in life. But prevention at any stage makes a difference." Therefore, everyone needs to be concerned about their risk of atherosclerosis. Knowing your blood pressure and LDL levels and, if necessary, making lifestyle changes can help reduce your chances of dying prematurely of heart disease.

Assignments

○ Read Chapter 12, "Cardiovascular Health," in Alters & Schiff, *Essential Concepts for Healthy Living*, 4th edition. You may find it helpful to take notes on your reading. Then read the Learning Objectives and Overview for this lesson. Review the Key Terms below.

○ Scan the Video Viewing Questions, and then watch the video program for Lesson 19, "Heart of the Matter."

○ After watching the video, answer the Video Viewing Questions and assess your learning with the Self-Test.

○ Complete the activities for Chapter 12 in the workbook that accompanies the textbook. Your instructor may use these activities as assignments.

Key Terms

The following terms and those defined in Chapter 12 of the textbook are important to your understanding of this unit.

aneurysm	— A swollen, weakened blood vessel.
angiogram	— An x-ray image of blood vessels after they have been injected with a contrast medium.
angioplasty	— The reconstruction of damaged blood vessels.
aorta	— The largest artery in the body.
CT scan (computerized tomography)	— A screening method in which thin, x-rayed sections of the body are reconstructed into three-dimensional images by a computer.
familial hypercholesterolemia	— Inherited condition characterized by very high blood cholesterol levels and increased risk of atherosclerosis.
MRI (magnetic resonance imaging)	— The use of magnetic fields and radio waves to visualize internal structures.
myocardial infarction	— Condition that occurs when an area of heart muscle dies because it does not receive enough oxygen. Medical term for heart attack.
restenosis	— Condition in which the abnormal narrowing of an artery recurs.

Video Viewing Questions

1. Dr. Hodis states, "...we're all at risk, and if [atherosclerosis is] in the family, a parent or sibling, then you're very high risk of also having...either stroke or heart disease." If people are in high-risk families, why should they be concerned about their cholesterol levels if they avoid tobacco products, get plenty of exercise, maintain healthy weights, eat low-cholesterol diets, and take other preventive measures?

2. What tests do physicians use to diagnose atherosclerosis? What procedures do physicians use to treat this condition?

3. What is the difference between HDL and LDL cholesterol? Why are high LDL levels a risk factor? What dietary and other lifestyle changes can people make to reduce their risk of atherosclerosis?

4. What are the signs and symptoms of heart attack, and how do they differ in men and women?

5. In families with a genetic predisposition to develop atherosclerosis, what lifestyle changes can young people make to reduce their risk?

Self-Test

Multiple Choice

1. Which of the following statements is true?
    a. Physicians use Pap tests to measure the width of the aorta.
    b. Atherectomy is a procedure that involves grafting leg veins into the heart.
    c. Iron accumulation in arteries is a sign of plaque formation.
    d. High levels of LDL cholesterol increase the risk of heart disease.

2. Rebecca has frequent bouts of anginal pain. What is causing her chest discomfort?
    a. Her heart muscle is not getting enough oxygen.
    b. Calcium deposits in her aorta are pressing on nerves in her chest.
    c. Plaque in her carotid arteries is blocking blood flow to her heart.
    d. She is having an allergic reaction to her nitroglycerin tablets.

3. According to Dr. Faxon, which of the following coronary care procedures is performed most often in the United States?
    a. Coronary appendectomy
    b. Ventricular stenosis diversion
    c. Balloon catheterization
    d. Coronary bypass procedure

4. Which of the following statements is false?
    a. Balloon angioplasty is an effective cure for coronary artery disease.
    b. Arterial plaques contain cholesterol.
    c. Surgeons can use lasers to remove small amounts of arterial plaque.
    d. Calcium deposits within arteries are often an indication of plaque build up.

5. Eric is 40 years old. He smokes cigarettes, is forty pounds overweight, and likes to watch television and surf the Internet. Eric's paternal grandfather had a fatal heart attack at age 49; his 65-year old father had a heart attack when Eric was 15 years old. You tell Eric that he cannot modify his
    a. cigarette smoking.
    b. family history.
    c. excess weight.
    d. lack of physical activity.

6. According to Dr. Sperling, which dietary program can decrease the risk of heart problems?
    a. High polyunsaturated, low fiber diet.
    b. Low saturated fat, low cholesterol diet.
    c. Low monounsaturated fat, high cholesterol diet.
    d. High saturated fat, high protein diet.

7. Which of the following statements is false?
   a. Cigarette smokers are more likely to develop cardiovascular disease than nonsmokers.
   b. Cigarette smokers can reduce their risk of heart disease by stopping smoking.
   c. Compounds in cigarette smoke increase arterial plaque formation.
   d. Cigarette smokers tend to have reduced LDL levels and increased HDL levels.

8. Why does a 45-year old man have a greater risk of heart attack than a 45-year old woman?
   a. Men are more ambitious and motivated to take dangerous risks than women.
   b. Job pressures and responsibilities are more stressful for men than for women.
   c. Women produce more estrogen, which protects them from heart disease until they reach menopause.
   d. Middle-aged women are less likely to smoke, be physically inactive, and eat high fat diets than middle-aged men.

Matching

Match the terms with the definitions that follow.

   a. angioplasty
   b. ischemia
   c. cardiac arrest
   d. aneurysm

____ 9. The heart stops beating

____ 10. Inadequate blood flow to tissues

____ 11. Weakened area of a blood vessel

____ 12. The reconstruction of damaged blood vessels

Short Answer

13. Although Jerry's total cholesterol level was 180 mg/dl of blood, he had a massive heart attack when he was 48 years old. Explain why total cholesterol may not provide a good indication of one's risk of cardiovascular disease.

14. Marissa has three severely blocked coronary arteries. Her physician suggests coronary bypass surgery. What would you tell Marissa about this procedure?

15. Samantha is 63 years old. She has a desk job, has mildly elevated blood pressure, is 20 pounds overweight, and smokes half a pack of cigarettes a day. She has no family history of atherosclerosis. Should she be concerned about her risk of atherosclerosis? Explain why or why not.

Expanded Analysis

1. According to Dr. Faxon, "Atherosclerosis...is a disease of childhood." What does he mean by this statement?

2. If one has a family history of dying from heart attack prematurely, why should this person modify his or her lifestyle?

3. Recently, physicians recognized that post-menopausal women are just as likely to die of heart disease as older men. Why do many women ignore their symptoms of heart disease?

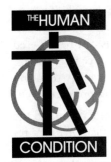

THE HUMAN
CONDITION

20

Brain Attack

Learning Objectives

Upon completing this lesson, you should be familiar with the facts, terms, and concepts presented in this lesson and should be able to:

○ List the major risk factors for stroke and the ages at which people are more susceptible.

○ Identify and differentiate between the two major types of strokes.

○ Describe the signs and symptoms of a stroke.

○ Explain why it is important to obtain prompt medical attention if a stroke is suspected.

○ Recognize the adaptability and responsiveness of the brain to rehabilitation efforts.

○ Designate attitudes and environments significant in achieving progress in stroke recovery.

Overview

Brain attack, or stroke, is the third leading cause of death in the United States. As they age, many Americans develop atherosclerosis, hardening and narrowing of the arteries. If a clot lodges in a narrowed artery that supplies the brain, it blocks the flow of blood. Without blood, brain cells will die within a few minutes, and the affected person experiences a stroke. Common causes of stroke include clots that clog the brain arteries and bleeding from the ruptured brain arteries.

Several risk factors for coronary artery disease, such as hypertension, high LDL cholesterol levels, and anxiety apply to stroke as well (see Table 12-2). People with hypertension have high risks of brain attacks. According to Dr. Saver, Neurology Director of the University of California–Los Angeles Stroke Center "...hypertension is the number one modifiable risk factor for stroke."

People often can reduce their risk of stroke by making lifestyle changes. High LDL cholesterol levels and physical inactivity increase the risk of hypertension. (See Table 12-3 for classifications of HDL and LDL levels.) By eating fewer fatty foods and exercising, LDL cholesterol levels can be lowered and HDL cholesterol levels raised. Exercise can also help reduce stress levels. Furthermore, many people with hypertension are salt-sensitive. By reducing their intake of salty foods, these people can lower their blood pressure levels.

Recently, scientists have added high blood levels of homocysteine to the list of risk factors for atherosclerosis. Certain dietary modifications may reduce elevated homocysteine levels, lowering the risk of stroke. The Consumer Health Box in Chapter 12 of your textbook describes the role of homocysteine in the development of atherosclerosis.

Detection and Treatment

The signs and symptoms of a stroke vary, but in most cases, one side of the body suddenly becomes weak, numb, or paralyzed. Additionally, brain attacks often impair speech and vision. Table 12-1 lists these and other signs and symptoms of stroke. If tissue plasminogen activator (tPA) is administered in the first few hours after the onset of a stroke, the individual may not experience serious and permanent brain damage. In some cases, however, surgery is needed to remove the clot that is placing pressure on the brain. Special brain imaging techniques such as MRIs and CAT scans help physicians identify the cause of stroke and locate affected areas of the brain.

Stroke recovery requires months of therapy. By practicing certain muscle movements, many patients are able to redevelop motor skills that had been performed effortlessly prior to the stroke. Such treatment enables healthy regions of the brain to participate in recovery by activating areas of the brain that were damaged. While observing MRI scans of a patient trying to move his paralyzed hand, Dr. Dobkin, Professor of Neurology at the University of California–Los Angeles notes that the patient uses both sides of his brain to move his hand, instead of using just one side, as he would normally do.

As seen in the cases of Karen Christensen and Jim Krakowski, rehabilitation takes time, practice, motivation, and perseverance. As Dr. Dobkin notes, "One of the terrific things about rehab is that it's not about being sick, it's about getting well...The key to rehabilitation...is to practice and practice those things that you want to do...."

Assignments

○ Review Chapter 12, "Cardiovascular Health," in Alters & Schiff, *Essential Concepts for Healthy Living*, 4th edition. You may find it helpful to take notes on your reading. Then read the Learning Objectives and Overview for this lesson. Review the Key Terms below.

○ Scan the Video Viewing Questions, and then watch the video program for Lesson 20, "Brain Attack."

○ After watching the video, answer the Video Viewing Questions and assess your learning with the Self-Test.

○ If you haven't done so already, complete the activities for Chapter 12 in the workbook that accompanies the textbook. Your instructor may use these activities as assignments.

Key Terms

The following terms and those defined in Chapter 12 of the textbook are important to your understanding of this unit.

atrial — Pertaining to the upper chambers of the heart, the atria.

diastolic pressure — The lower number in the blood pressure reading.

epidemiologic — Pertaining to the study of the causation, occurrence, and distribution of illness in a population.

homocysteine — A by product of normal protein metabolism that may damage arteries.

ischemia — Decreased blood supply to an organ, body part, or tissue.

systolic pressure — The higher number in the blood pressure reading.

tissue plasminogen activator (tPA) — A drug that breaks up blood clots.

Video Viewing Questions

1. What happens when a stroke occurs? What are major risk factors for stroke?

2. Dr. Saver, Neurology Director at the University of Southern California-Los Angeles Stroke Center, mentions several lifestyle steps that people can take to reduce their risk of stroke. What are these steps?

3. What are the symptoms of stroke? According to Dr. Saver, how should you respond if you think you or someone you know may be having a stroke?

4. What is the "window for intervention" for acute stroke?

5. How are physicians using newer diagnostic and treatment methods to diagnose and treat stroke? How can these technological advances help stroke patients?

6. What can be done during stroke recovery to reduce the risk of complications and regain physical functioning?

Self-Test

Multiple Choice

1. Which of the following statements is true?
    a. Stroke occurs when excessive neurotransmitters are released into brain synapses.
    b. Stroke is the second leading cause of death for Americans.
    c. People who are middle-aged and older have the highest risk of stroke.
    d. If your diastolic pressure is between 60 and 84, you should try to lower it.

2. The "silent killer" is
    a. heart attack.
    b. high blood pressure.
    c. diverticular disease.
    d. diabetes mellitus.

3. Your latest blood pressure measurement was normal. Which of the following blood pressure measurements could have been yours?
    a. 190/100
    b. 170/85
    c. 120/70
    d. 60/90

4. Which of the following tests is used to determine the extent of a stroke?
    a. EKG
    b. Pap
    c. PSA
    d. MRI

5. When a clot partially blocks the flow of blood to a part of the brain, an _____ attack occurs.
    a. ischemic
    b. emetic
    c. anemic
    d. osmotic

6. Amy's physicians suspect she's had a stroke. Which of the following signs or symptoms would you expect Amy to have?
    a. Paralysis on her left side
    b. Loud rapid speech
    c. Painfully swollen joints
    d. Spotty rectal bleeding

7. After Jim had a stroke, his therapy included maintaining an upright position. Such treatment reduces the risk of
    a. full recovery.
    b. gravity infusion.
    c. supine psychosis.
    d. pressure sores.

118

Match the terms with the definitions that follow.

    a. tPA
    b. diastolic
    c. systolic
    d. ischemia

____   8. Condition that occurs when blood flow is interrupted

____   9. Clot-busting drug

____ 10. Top number in blood pressure reading

____ 11. Bottom number in blood pressure reading

12. Your physician reports that your blood pressure is "a little high," and she recommends that you make some lifestyle changes to lower it. What recommendations would you expect to receive from your physician?

13. Your best friend's father suddenly complains of having difficulty seeing. You think he might be having a stroke. Discuss what you should do to help.

14. Phyllis is a 25-year-old woman who had a stroke during the 36th week of pregnancy. While she was hospitalized, physicians delivered her baby. A couple of weeks later, Phyllis' 75-year-old grandfather had a stroke. Both individuals underwent the same rehabilitation program. After six months, Phyllis has regained almost all physical and cognitive functioning, but her grandfather is having difficulty walking and talking. Explain why Phyllis recovered faster.

Expanded Analysis

1. Does your lifestyle increase your risk of stroke? Discuss lifestyle modifications that you can make to reduce your risk.

2. Dr. Dobkin refers to the "...plasticity or adaptability of the brain...." What does he mean? How does the plasticity or adaptability of the brain enable a stroke patient to recover some of the functional abilities lost when his or her brain was damaged by the lack of oxygen?

3. According to Dr. Dobkin, the key to rehabilitation is practice. In addition to practicing physical activities, what other factors increase the likelihood that one will recover partially or completely from a stroke?

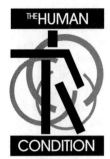

THE HUMAN
CONDITION

21

diagnosis: Cancer

Learning Objectives

Upon completing this lesson, you should be familiar with the facts, terms, and concepts presented in the lesson and should be able to:

○ Define cancer and describe the circumstances within cells that give rise to the disease.

○ Recognize the risk factors for major cancers, and how they can be "managed" or reduced.

○ Be aware of the warning signals for cancer and the importance of early detection.

○ Give examples of screening tests and techniques used to identify major forms of cancer.

○ Explain how epidemiological data help scientists isolate the causes of cancer.

Overview

Today, the diagnosis of cancer is not an automatic death sentence. Although cancer is the second leading cause of death in the United States, many cancers can be cured, especially if detected early. Cancer prevention, however, remains a major public health concern. As scientists learn more about the biological processes that cause cancer, effective preventive measures may become available.

Cancer is not a single disease, but the general name for over 100 different diseases. All cancers, however, have common characteristics: cancer cells exhibit abnormal growth, division, and differentiation. Unlike normal cells that stop growing and dividing at appropriate times, cancer cells grow and divide unchecked. These cells may form masses called malignant tumors, which interfere with the functioning of tissues and organs. Cancer cells also have the ability to spread (metastasize) from where they develop. Once the cancer has metastasized, it is more difficult to control.

121

Only cells that have certain damaged genes (mutations) become cancerous. Oncogenes are mutated genes that act like "on switches" to enable the cell to grow faster than normal. Cells also have tumor-suppressor genes that act as "off switches" to slow cellular growth. When tumor-suppressor genes mutate, they no longer limit cell growth. Therefore, cancer results from an activation of oncogenes and deactivation of tumor-suppressor genes.

According to Dr. Varmus, former Director of the National Institutes of Health, "Human cancer is a genetic disease in an unusual way. Some altered genes are inherited, but that's an uncommon event. Much more commonly, our genes undergo changes in only a few cells during the course of our lifetime. And certain constellations of changes predispose a cell [to] becoming a runaway…a maverick cell that we know is a cancer cell."

Although heredity plays a role in the transmission of faulty genes that result in cancer, only five to ten percent of all cancers are thought to be inherited. Lifestyle and environmental factors contribute to the development of most cancers by causing mutations. So the key to cancer prevention involves changing one's lifestyle and environment.

The results of experimental and epidemiological studies indicate that mutations are caused by exposure to carcinogens, such as certain drugs, low-dose radiation, and toxic chemicals. Cancer often has a long natural history; that is, the disease develops years, even decades after exposure to a carcinogen. Therefore, the chance of developing most cancers increases as one ages. Understanding which environmental hazard or exposure produces cancer-causing mutations can help researchers determine how lifestyle can be altered to reduce the risk of cancer.

Being at risk for cancer, however, doesn't mean that one automatically develops the disease. Furthermore, being free of risk factors doesn't mean one is immune from cancer. As seen in the video episode, Cynthia Lauren followed a healthy lifestyle and had no family history of breast cancer, yet developed the disease at an early age.

Although one cannot change some cancer risk factors, such as heredity, age, race, and ethnicity; other risk factors, such as smoking, obesity, and excessive exposure to sunlight, can be avoided. Scientific discoveries indicate that smoking is a major risk factor for lung and many other cancers. According to Dr. Glaspy of the Jonsson Comprehensive Cancer Center at the University of California–Los Angeles, society has failed to translate the information concerning the hazards of smoking into effective and socially acceptable prevention strategies. Despite public health efforts to "spread the word," too many people still are smoking and still developing lung cancer.

What can we expect from cancer research in this century? Until researchers have a better understanding of what causes cancer, a cure or effective form of prevention is not likely. Although Dr. Ganz, Director of the Division of Cancer Prevention and Control Research at the Jonsson Comprehensive Cancer Center, thinks that it may not be possible to eradicate all cancers, it will be possible to "…somehow modify that risk [of cancer] and actually prevent the disease from occurring."

Assignments

○ Read Chapter 13, "Cancer," in Alters & Schiff, *Essential Concepts for Healthy Living*, 4th edition. You may find it helpful to take notes on your reading. Then read the Learning Objectives and Overview for this lesson. Review the Key Terms below.

◯ Scan the Video Viewing Questions, and then watch the video program for Lesson 21, "diagnosis: Cancer."

◯ After watching the video, answer the Video Viewing Questions and assess your learning with the Self-Test.

◯ Complete the activities for Chapter 13 in the workbook that accompanies the textbook. Your instructor may use these activities as a assignments.

Key Terms

The following terms and those defined in Chapter 13 of the textbook are important to your understanding of this unit.

benign tumors — Encapsulated masses of cells that remain in one location and do not invade surrounding tissues.

biopsy — A small piece of tissue that is taken from a growth so that the cells can be studied and a diagnosis confirmed.

colonoscopy — A procedure in which a physician views the entire length of the colon using a flexible fiber-optic tube.

epidemiology — Study of the causation, occurrence, and distribution of illness in a population.

hypothesis — A tentative explanation or prediction.

malignant tumors — Masses of cancer cells that invade body tissues and interfere with the normal functioning of tissues and organs.

mutations — Changes in genes or chromosomes; damaged genes.

nasopharyngeal — The region of the throat that is behind the nose and extends into the windpipe.

oncogenes — Tumor genes that manufacture altered proteins, which speed cell growth and decrease the level of cell differentiation.

Papanicolaou test (Pap test) — A screening procedure for cervical cancer in which cells from the cervical canal are removed and then smeared on a glass slide for microscopic examination.

risk factors — Conditions that, when present, increase the chances that a person will develop a particular disease.

second-hand smoke — The passive inhalation, by nonsmokers, of environmental tobacco smoke present in the air.

tumor-suppressor genes— Genes that slow cell growth.

Video Viewing Questions

1. As Dr. Varmus states, "Human cancer is a genetic disease in an unusual way…some altered genes are inherited, but that's an uncommon event. Much more commonly our genes undergo…certain constellations of changes [that] predispose [a cell to] becoming a runaway – a maverick cell that we know is a cancer cell." What are some of the factors that cause the development of these runaway cells?

2. Dr. Ganz counsels women who are at high risk for breast cancer. What are some of the risk factors that Dr. Ganz uses to estimate a woman's risk of this disease?

3. Early detection is a key factor in surviving a cancer diagnosis. The earlier cancer is diagnosed and treated, the better the chance of survival. What are some of the most useful methods of cancer detection?

4. There are many recommendations concerning what can be done to prevent cancer. What significant lifestyle changes can a person make to reduce his or her risk of cancer?

5. When comparing cancer rates and incidences within certain regions and populations, different patterns become evident. For example, breast, lung, colon, and prostate cancers commonly affect populations living in more highly developed nations; liver, cervical, and esophageal cancers are more prevalent in populations living in less developed countries and Asia. How can epidemiologists use this information?

6. According to Dr. Glaspy and Dr. Ganz, what new developments in cancer prevention and risk reduction can be expected in the next five to twenty years?

Self-Test

Multiple Choice

1. A cell in the large intestine undergoes changes that indicate it is preparing to divide into two cells. What controls the timing and events of this change?
   a. Hereditary material
   b. Primary isoflavones
   c. Maintenance factors
   d. Regular vitamins

2. Phil is a chemist for a pharmaceutical company. For years he's been using benzene to extract certain compounds from plants that might have medicinal value. Although Phil has been careful while working with benzene, some of the chemical has gotten onto his hands. Recently, Phil developed a sore on his left hand that wouldn't heal. After examining the sore, Phil's doctor told him that it is a form of skin cancer, resulting from years of contact with benzene. Which of the following terms describes benzene?
   a. An oncogene
   b. A tumor stimulator
   c. A malignant activator
   d. A carcinogen

3. Recently, Helena noticed blood in her bowel movements. She is worried about her risk of colon cancer because her father died from the disease. To screen Helena for cancer of the colon and rectum, her physician should perform a
   a. fiberoptic examination.
   b. gamma test.
   c. bariatric measurement.
   d. Pap test.

4. Ricky has a cancerous tumor in his left lung. A CT scan indicates that the cancer has metastasized. This means that the cancer cells have:
   a. expanded, enlarging the size of the primary tumor.
   b. spread from Ricky's lung to other organs.
   c. undergone a transformation and have become benign.
   d. disappeared, and Ricky is free of the disease.

5. Which of the following women has a higher than normal risk of breast cancer?
   a. A woman who smokes cigarettes.
   b. A woman who had her first menstrual period when she was 15 years old.
   c. A woman who exercises nearly every day.
   d. A woman who produces more estrogen than an average woman.

6. If Americans would make one lifestyle change, the number of cancer deaths would drop dramatically over the next 50 years. That change would be to
   a. eat less meat.
   b. drink less alcohol.
   c. stop smoking.
   d. take more vitamins.

Match the terms with the definitions that follow.   **Matching**
   a. malignant
   b. dysplasia
   c. benign
   d. carcinogen
   e. biopsy

_____ 7. The removal of a small piece of tissue for diagnosing cancer

_____ 8. A cell that is not cancerous

_____ 9. A cancer-causing substance

_____ 10. A cell that is cancerous

_____ 11. A cell that has the potential to become cancerous

12. Discuss how cancer results from mutations.   **Short Answer**

13. Cynthia Lauren's breast cancer was detected at a relatively advanced stage; stage III. Discuss the importance of detecting cancer in its early stages.

14. Epidemiological studies provide information about patterns of disease distribution within populations. Using cancer as an example, explain how medical researchers use this information.

Expanded Analysis

1. Teams of researchers in China and the United States investigate whether long-term exposure to a certain chemical increases the risk of skin cancer. Although the Chinese researchers find such an association, U.S. researchers do not find that long-term exposure to the chemical increases the risk of skin cancer. What factors could explain why the two teams of researchers obtained these very different findings?

2. Do you know anyone with cancer? If so, what type of cancer? How was the disease diagnosed? Do you think this person's lifestyle was a factor in the development of the disease? If so, which high risk behavior(s) may have contributed to the development of the cancer? How did the diagnosis change this person's life?

3. Throughout the world and even within a country, rates and types of cancer vary. How can epidemiologists use information concerning patterns of cancer occurrence within a region or population to determine risk factors? In your answer, give an example of a type of cancer that does not occur to the same extent in various populations.

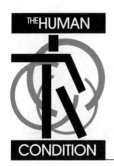

22

Living with Cancer

Learning Objectives

Upon completing this lesson, you should be familiar with the facts and concepts presented in this lesson and should be able to:

○ Explain why many medical professionals consider cancer a chronic disease.

○ Compare the three traditional forms of cancer treatment, how they are used individually, and how they are used in conjunction with each other.

○ Recognize the concepts behind some of the newer approaches to cancer treatment.

○ Examine the use of clinical trials in developing new treatment modalities to fight various forms of cancer.

○ Discuss the value of support groups for cancer victims.

Overview

Not long ago, people with cancer had few treatment options. Today, advances in technology and scientific research have increased the number and effectiveness of therapies so that many forms of the disease are curable. Nevertheless, a diagnosis of cancer still frightens people. In addition to facing the possibility of dying prematurely, many patients must make difficult decisions concerning their treatment. Breast cancer survivor Cynthia Lauren recalls her reaction to the diagnosis: "...I had to deal with being stunned and afraid, and I had to learn, so I could make the best choices for myself."

Cancer affects more than the patient's physical health. Enduring the disease and its treatments can damage the patient's psychological, social, and spiritual health, too. Additionally, the diagnosis of cancer often exacts a heavy toll on family members and friends. Enlisting their support, however, can provide another weapon for the patient to use against this terrible disease.

The principal forms of cancer treatment are surgery, chemotherapy, and radiation. Surgical procedures involve removal of some healthy tissue along with the cancerous tumor to increase the likelihood that no malignant cells remain. Since cancer cells may have spread beyond the original tumor site, can-

Controlling
Cancer

cer specialists often use chemotherapy and radiation treatment in addition to surgery. Chemotherapy is the use of drugs to destroy cancer cells or inhibit their ability to reproduce. Radiation therapies kill malignant cells by targeting them with high doses of radiation.

Experimental forms of treatment include gene therapy, angiogenesis-inhibiting drugs, and biomodulation (immunotherapy). Gene therapy involves using special viruses to replace the damaged genetic material of cancer cells with healthy genetic information. Angiogenesis-inhibiting drugs interfere with the blood supply to tumors, killing malignant cells. Biomodulation is the manipulation of the body's own immune system to rid itself of cancer.

Scientists have discovered that the malignant cells of certain breast cancers contain antigens that act as "antennae," receiving and relaying information to the cell's nucleus. Such information is necessary for the cancer cell's growth and survival. Recently, researchers developed Herceptin, an antibody that selectively binds to these antigens, rendering them nonfunctional. Herceptin does not affect normal cells.

Before Herceptin or any other new cancer-fighting drugs can be made available for general use, researchers conduct clinical trials involving cancer patients to determine their effectiveness. Based on the results of these studies, a drug may get approval from the Food and Drug Administration (FDA) for use as an anticancer drug. Harold Varmus, the former Director of the National Institutes of Health and former chief of the Varmus Laboratory at the National Cancer Research Institute, says, "...clinical trials that involve patients with cancer have made extraordinary contributions to our treatment of cancer." Because most American children with cancer are enrolled in clinical trials, many childhood cancers have effective treatments. Few adults, however, participate in such studies.

Although the results of clinical trials often indicate that a treatment is effective, they may also show that the treatment causes serious side effects that must be considered by the patient. Tamoxifen is a good example of a drug that prevents breast cancer, but its use increases the risk of endometrial cancer. Dr. Leslie Bernstein, Professor of Preventive Medicine at the University of Southern California, points out that the risk of developing breast cancer is far greater than the risk of endometrial cancer. The patient must weigh tamoxifen's risks and benefits before undergoing treatment.

Psychological Aspects

Living with cancer affects the patient's physical health, but the experience also affects psychological, social, and spiritual aspects of his or her health and well-being. An important way that the patient can cope with the concerns and problems associated with cancer is to discuss the experience with others. Some cancer patients have found that joining support groups is helpful. Support groups provide an opportunity for patients to share experiences and educate others about the disease and its treatments.

In addition to finding comfort from others in support groups, many people living with cancer obtain emotional support from family members. Dr. Ganz, Director of the Division of Cancer Prevention and Control Research at the Jonsson Comprehensive Cancer Center at the University of California–Los Angeles, says "...cancer is a family disease." When a loved one has cancer, the disease affects the person's family too. Children are especially hard hit when a parent has the disease. Communication between and among family members can help ease their concerns and fears. Family members can assist the patient in many ways, but perhaps most importantly by providing much needed encouragement and moral support.

For many people living with cancer, the diagnosis provides them with an opportunity to examine their lives closely and decide what is truly important. By doing so, these people are able to make something positive out of a life-threatening experience. Living with cancer profoundly affects their lives. As Dr. Coscarelli points out, "…those women in there were very invested in life. They were invested in living, and they were invested in taking this cancer experience, which is extraordinarily difficult, and they wanted to turn it into something good."

Assignments

○ Review Chapter 13, "Cancer," in Alters & Schiff, *Essential Concepts for Healthy Living*, 4th edition. You may find it helpful to take notes on your reading. Then read the Learning Objectives and Overview for this lesson. Review the Key Terms below.

○ Scan the Video Viewing Questions, and then watch the video program for Lesson 22, "Living With Cancer."

○ After watching the video, answer the Video Viewing Questions and assess your learning with the Self-Test.

○ If you haven't done so already, complete the activities for Chapter 13 in the workbook that accompanies the textbook. Your instructor may use these activities and assignments.

Key Terms

The following terms and those defined in Chapter 13 of the textbook are important to your understanding of this unit.

angiogenesis	— The ability to stimulate the development of blood vessels.
antibody	— A protein that binds to substances that might harm the body, rendering them ineffective.
biomodulation	— Treatments that manipulate the body's immune system, enhancing its response to cancerous cells; immunotherapies.
chemotherapy	— Cancer treatment involving the use of drugs; "chemo."
clinical trials	— Research involving human subjects that determines the safety and effectiveness of drugs.
efficacy	— The ability of a drug or treatment to produce a result; effectiveness.
endometrial	— Pertaining to the endometrium, the lining of the uterus.
lumpectomy	— Surgical removal of a breast tumor, including a layer of surrounding tissue.

placebo	— A sham treatment that is used to determine the effectiveness of experimental treatments.
proton therapy	— A form of radiation treatment that uses a stream of positively-charged, subatomic particles to kill cancerous cells.
modified radical mastectomy	— The surgical removal of a breast, underarm fat and lymph nodes without the removal of underlying muscle; one treatment for breast cancer.
radical mastectomy	— The surgical removal of a breast, underlying muscle tissue, and underarm fat and lymph nodes; one treatment for breast cancer.
mastectomy	— The surgical removal of a breast to treat breast cancer.

Video Viewing Questions

1. Cancer treatment often causes side effects. For example, conventional cancer treatments usually destroy some healthy tissue along with cancerous tissue. How do newer treatments such as proton therapy and gene therapy reduce this damage?

2. How are the results of clinical trials used to improve cancer treatments?

3. Dr. Ganz says, "…statistics…can give [patients] a very accurate appraisal of their likely benefit or their risks for taking certain treatments." When discussing tamoxifen, Dr. Bernstein says, "…we then want to weigh the risks and the benefits." What are these physicians referring to when they mention risks and benefits?

4. Dr. Coscarelli points out that, "…relationships become affected as people react to the diagnosis…and share in that experience." When one has cancer, how can the disease affect friends and family?

5. Ann, a woman in the support group, says, "I think one of the things that happened with me is that cancer became rephrased into something that was normal…you are alive, you have cancer…you continue." What does she mean?

Self-Test

Multiple Choice

1. Jean has been diagnosed with breast cancer. She found the pea-sized lump in her breast early, before it had metastasized. She has many choices to make concerning treatment. Her physician will probably recommend that she undergo _____ before other treatments.

    a. acupuncture

    b. lumpectomy

    c. mutation therapy

    d. placebo therapy

2. Leanna has breast cancer. The results of blood tests indicate that she has abnormal HER2/NEU genes. Her physician is likely to recommend that the cancer be treated with
    a. herceptin.
    b. radiotherapy.
    c. acupuncture.
    d. biopsy.

3. About 30 percent of the participants in a clinical trial of a new anticancer drug report having more energy while taking the medication. These people, however, are taking pills that contain no chemicals that would affect the body. This finding indicates that the treatment is a
    a. placebo.
    b. chemotherapy.
    c. biomodulator.
    d. stimulant.

4. Before a new anticancer drug can be marketed, it needs the approval of which federal agency?
    a. The Federal Drug Management Commission
    b. The Bureau of Chemical Applications
    c. The Drug Enforcement Administration
    d. The Food and Drug Administration

5. An experimental cancer treatment that uses viruses to convey information that may change the DNA of malignant cells is
    a. proton therapy.
    b. mutation therapy.
    c. gene therapy.
    d. Antimalignancy therapy.

6. Which of the following studies is used to determine the safety and effectiveness of anticancer drugs?
    a. Clinical trials
    b. Epidemiological research
    c. Anecdotal evidence
    d. Pharmacological surveys

7. A physician treats Ken's cancerous tumor by giving him antibodies that bind to antigens on cancer cell membranes. This treatment is a form of
    a. lumpectomy.
    b. immunotherapy.
    c. mutation therapy.
    d. angiogenesis therapy.

8. Which of the following treatments stops the growth of a cancerous tumor by cutting off its blood supply?
    a. Proton therapy
    b. Gene therapy
    c. Angiogenesis-inhibiting therapy
    d. Herceptin therapy

Matching

Match the terms with the definitions that follow.
a. mastectomy
b. chemotherapy
c. proton therapy
d. biomodulation

_____ 9. Surgical removal of the breast to treat breast cancer

_____ 10. Form of radiation therapy to treat cancer

_____ 11. Use of anticancer drugs

_____ 12. Use of body's immune system to treat cancer

Short Answer

13. How does Herceptin interfere with the growth of cancer cells, yet spare normal cells?

14. Explain the value of testing drugs in clinical trials.

15. Discuss the benefits of support groups for cancer patients.

Expanded Analysis

1. How do you think you would react if you were diagnosed with cancer? How do you think the diagnosis would affect your family? Would you want to join a support group? Why or why not?

2. When cancer affects an older adult and grows slowly, cancer specialists may use a "wait and see" form of treatment that involves no specific therapies other than keeping watch over the progress of the disease. After viewing "Living with Cancer," why do you think this form of treatment may be more desirable than surgery, chemotherapy or radiation treatment?

3. Why are placebos used in clinical trials? If a patient responds positively to a placebo, explain why you think the patient's physician should or should not inform the patient about the treatment.

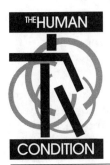

23

Age Happens

Learning Objectives

Upon completing this lesson, you should be familiar with the facts and concepts presented in this lesson and should be able to:

○ Distinguish physiological changes associated with the normal aging process from those changes that are not normal aspects of growing old.

○ Discuss the effects that aging can have on health and well being.

○ Explain what is meant by "successful aging."

○ Suggest behaviors that increase a person's chances of living a long and healthy life.

○ Compare independent living and assisted living options for older adults.

Overview

Aging is a pattern of changes that naturally occurs as one grows older. Dean Hamer, Chief of Gene Structure & Regulation, National Cancer Institute, National Institutes of Health, compares the human body to an American car: "…as we grow older, our parts begin to wear out, in essence, we begin to rust." Of course, we don't actually "rust," but our bodies do show the effects of time and begin to wear out. However, taking good care of your body can increase your life expectancy just as taking good car of a car can extend its mileage.

Many of the physical changes that the human body undergoes as it ages are normal and should be expected. These changes include menopause in women, decrease in blood circulation, graying and thinning hair, wrinkles, loss of height, reduced muscle mass, loss of muscular strength, declining metabolic rate, and loss of near vision (presbyopia). Several of the physical conditions that people often associate with aging are not normal. For example, osteoarthritis and osteoporosis affect many older adults, but these chronic conditions are not normal. Table 15-1 in the textbook lists normal physiological changes associated with aging.

Aging: Normal or Abnormal?

Today, about 12 percent of the U.S. population is at least 65 years of age. This segment of the population is growing faster than younger segments, because the "Baby Boom" generation of Americans is living longer. Today, it is not difficult to find Americans who are at least 100 years old. According to the U.S. Census Bureau, 4 million Americans will be more than 100 years of age by 2050.

At this point, there are no pills or potions that one can take to guarantee longevity. Heredity, however, can provide an important key to longevity. As Dr. Hamer notes, "People that have long-lived parents are more likely to live a long life." Nevertheless, environment and lifestyle also influence the aging process and longevity. By adopting healthier lifestyles, young people increase their chances of aging successfully. People who age successfully are not affected substantially by the usual physical changes and loss of body functions that are associated with growing old. According to Dr. Mosqueda, Director of Geriatrics at University of California–Irvine, Medical Center, "Things that help people age successfully are things that our moms probably taught us. Eat right, exercise, stay involved and active."

Eating a nutritious diet, getting regular exercise, and engaging in intellectually stimulating activities are necessary for enjoying a long and healthy life. Frail, elderly women who live alone are at risk of malnutrition because they often make poor food choices. As one ages, exercise continues to be important for maintaining good health. Some physical activities, however, are unsuitable for elderly people. Appropriate exercises are those that most elderly people can perform easily, comfortably and without the need for special facilities. According to Dr. Lipson, Chief of the Division of Geriatric Medicine, University of Southern California, walking is an excellent physical activity for many elderly people.

People who age successfully are not only physically healthy but also involved in a variety of intellectually stimulating activities. Regardless of age, feeling useful and being productive are necessary for preserving a high level of self-esteem and sense of well-being.

Unhealthy Aging

Before they reach age 65, many people develop chronic conditions, such as diabetes and heart disease, that reduce longevity. Through proper diet and regular exercise, a person with diabetes can often control the damaging effects of the disease. Many people with diabetes, however, do not take good care of themselves, and over time, the disease causes serious complications, such as nerve and blood vessel damage. If poorly controlled, diabetes contributes to heart disease, stroke, and circulatory problems that can result in loss of lower limbs.

Millions of aging Americans suffer from some form of arthritis and osteoporosis. Arthritis is a broad group of joint diseases characterized by degeneration of the cartilage. Cartilage protects the ends of bones where they meet in joints. Arthritis causes painfully swollen and inflamed joints. Most elderly people have some osteoarthritis, the most common form of arthritis. This chronic condition probably results from years of wear and tear on weight-bearing joints, such as those in the knees, hands, feet, and hips. Osteoporosis, thinning of the bones, can result in fractures. Hip fractures are a major threat to elderly persons; many people with such injuries die or are disabled permanently. Dr. Lipson notes, "...by age 90, one in three...[Caucasian women] will have had a broken hip, and during the acute process of the hip fracture, one in three will die."

As they age, many adults fear that they are showing early signs of Alzheimer's disease when they forget a relative's birthday or where they placed their eyeglasses. Everyone experiences some minor lapses of memory as they grow older, but according to Dr. Mosqueda, "…significant memory loss is not a normal change of aging." Memory loss that is associated with losses of other areas of cognitive functioning is called dementia. Age-related dementias, such as Alzheimer's disease, are a progressive loss of cognitive functioning that affects about 10 percent of the population who are over 65 years of age. The inability to recognize one's children, acknowledge where one is living, recall the date, count backwards from 20, or make rational decisions are signs of dementia. Age-related dementia is the major reason for placing people into nursing homes, because people suffering from these conditions are unable to live independently and their care can be burdensome to spouses or other family members.

Although Alzheimer's disease is incurable, medications can control some of the behaviors. Other conditions, which may be treatable, can mimic Alzheimer's disease. For example, stroke and overmedication (polypharmacy) produce losses of cognitive functioning that may be misdiagnosed as Alzheimer's disease. Although there is no cure for Alzheimer's disease, the loss of normal cognition that occurs with overmedication is usually reversible when the medications are withdrawn. Therefore, it is important to determine the cause when loss of cognitive functioning is observed in an older adult.

Assisted Living

Many older adults reach a point at which they need some degree of assistance with daily tasks. Jennifer Devoll, Director of Admissions at Hollenbeck Home, says assisted living "…can be something as simple as helping people with their medicines and providing transportation to their doctor's appointments…It can be assistance with bathing…dressing, [and] reminder services…."

Some centers such as the Over 60 Health Center in East Oakland, California, provide a variety of such services to assist elderly people who still reside in their homes. These services enable healthy older adults to function independently for longer periods. Dr. Mosqueda says, "The number one fear of older adults is loss of independence."

For elderly people who are no longer able to take care of themselves in their own homes, moving into an assisted living care facility is an option. In these residential facilities, the older adult can get help with transportation needs, bathing, dressing, or feeding. Hollenbeck Home, for example, provides aging residents with nutritious meals, physical activities, and social and intellectual stimulation in a home-like atmosphere. These features are vital for maintaining the health and well-being of elderly people.

As in a younger person, a strong social support network can help the aged individual cope with life's crises. Dr. Lipson says, "Sometimes congregate living may be more healthy than just living by yourself…. If you stay by yourself, you become sort of like a hermit…you lose social skills and relevance." Although residing in residential facilities such as Hollenbeck Home requires major adjustments on the part of the elderly person, congregate living often enables the resident to feel secure, enjoy the benefits of a strong social support network, and be creative and productive.

Assignments

○ Read Chapter 15, "Aging, Dying, and Death," in Alters & Schiff, *Essential Concepts for Healthy Living*, 4th edition, paying particular attention to pages 423–433. You may find it helpful to take notes on your reading. Then read the Learning Objectives and Overview for this lesson. Review the Key Terms below.

○ Scan the Video Viewing Questions, and then watch the video program for Lesson 23, "Age Happens."

○ After watching the video, answer the Video Viewing Questions and assess your learning with the Self-Test.

○ Complete the activities for Chapter 15 in the workbook that accompanies the textbook. Your instructor may use these activities as assignments.

Key Terms

The following terms and those defined in Chapter 15 are important to your understanding of this unit.

aging	— The sum of all changes that occur in an organism over its life span.
arthritis	— A group of diseases characterized by pain, stiffness and inflammation of the joints.
cognitive	— Pertaining to mental processes that include memory, reasoning and awareness of surroundings.
congregate living	— A type of housing in which a person or family has private living quarters but shares a common dining room and other facilities with other members of the community.
life span	— The maximum number of years that members of a particular species can expect to live when conditions are optimal.
polypharmacy	— The side effects of taking too much or too many medications; overmedication.

Video Viewing Questions

1. Dr. Hamer compares the human body to a car. Using this analogy, what does he mean by "planned obsolescence?" Which physiological changes are associated with normal aging and which are associated with disease processes?

2. Dr. Hamer states, "…aging and dying, like many aspects of our health, are at least partly controlled by our genes." How does heredity contribute to longevity? Since people cannot choose their parents, what can they do to increase their chances of living a long and healthy life?

3. A key to successful aging is exercise. Which factors need to be considered when choosing appropriate exercises for an older adult? According to Dr. Lipson, which physical activity is suitable for most elderly people?

4. What is osteoarthritis, and what causes this condition? What is osteoporosis, and why is it such a serious threat to elderly people?

5. What distinguishes the loss of memory that occurs with normal aging from that which occurs in age-related dementia? Besides the dementia that results from Alzheimer's disease, what other conditions produce similar losses of cognition?

6. What does Dr. Lipson mean when he says, "Sometimes congregate living may be more healthy than just living by yourself…" What is "assisted living"?

Self-Test

Multiple Choice

1. According to the video, what percentage of the American population is 65 years of age and older?
   a. 2 percent
   b. 12 percent
   c. 22 percent
   d. 32 percent

2. Which of the following changes or conditions is associated with the normal aging process?
   a. reduced muscular strength
   b. osteoarthritis
   c. faster reaction times
   d. increased metabolism

3. In the ten years after menopause, Betty lost 2 inches in height. Her upper back is curved, forming a hump. Last week she fell and broke her hip. A bone density test indicated that her bones are brittle. Her condition is probably the result of
   a. osteomalacia.
   b. osteoporosis.
   c. osteoarthritis.
   d. osteomyelitis.

4. Duncan is 78 years old. For several years, he has been taking 2 pills for his heart, but a month ago, the doctor prescribed 2 more medicines to control Duncan's diabetes and depression. Lately, his wife reports that he has been forgetting things that just happened. Yesterday, he drove his

car through the garage door. Which of the following conditions is the most likely explanation for his unusual behavior?

a. Duncan is just displaying normal changes associated with the aging process.

b. Duncan is just too busy and has too many things on his mind.

c. Duncan is showing signs of polypharmacy.

d. Duncan is acting forgetful and destroying property to get his wife's attention.

5. According to Dr. Lipson, which of the following physical activities would be suitable for most older adults?

a. horseback riding

b. bicycling

c. jogging

d. mall walking

6. Darrel had excellent vision until his 45th birthday, when he noticed that he couldn't read his birthday cards unless he held them at arm's length away from his face. Darrel probably has

a. glaucoma.

b. cataracts.

c. presbyopia.

d. incontinence.

7. Betty is 63 years old. When she wakes up in the morning, the joints of her fingers are painfully stiff and her knees hurt. She probably has

a. osteoarthritis.

b. osteoporosis.

c. incontinence.

d. rheumatic fever.

8. Which of the following statements is false?

a. Alzheimer's disease is incurable.

b. Alzheimer's is a normal feature of growing old.

c. The symptoms of Alzheimer's disease can occur during middle age.

d. Using aluminum cookware does not cause Alzheimer's disease.

9. Which of the following conditions is a major cause of memory loss in elderly people?

a. Osteoporosis

b. Arthritis

c. Incontinence

d. Strokes

10. Which of the following statements is true?

a. A major fear of aging people is losing their independence.

b. Dementia occurs when the heart pumps more blood with each beat.

c. After 65 years of age, the brain increases in size and weight.

d. Judo and bicycling are suitable activities for older adults with arthritis in their hips.

Short Answer

11. Explain how heredity influences longevity. Using an example, discuss how lifestyle affects the aging process.

12. You have a job assisting the activities director at an assisted care facility. Discuss factors you should consider when choosing appropriate exercises for the residents.

13. Maria, who takes care of her 82-year-old mother, worries that her mother has Alzheimer's disease. Although you suggest that Maria take her mother to see a physician for a complete check-up, Maria asks you for more information about the disease. Discuss what you would tell Maria.

Expanded Analysis

1. Discuss what you like least about the aging process. Are there aspects of growing old that you think are positive? Explain why.

2. When describing older adults, Jennifer Devoll says, "…they really are just people. Like people of any age, they are just all different personalities, and they have all different traits and quirks…They're just individuals." How did you feel toward older adults or the aging process before watching the video? Were your feelings stereotypical? Did your feelings change after watching "Age Happens"?

3. What impressed you the most about Hollenbeck Home and its residents? Would you want to live in a similar community when you are over 75 years old? What would be the pros and cons of living in an assisted living facility?

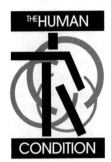

24

Final Chapter

Learning Objectives

Upon completing this lesson, you should be familiar with the facts and concepts presented in the lesson and should be able to:

○ Explain the value of having an advance directive.

○ Discuss the five stages that Kübler-Ross developed to describe the emotional response of dying persons.

○ Recognize changes that are occurring within the medical profession in response to demands for patient self-determination and palliative care.

○ Define euthanasia and differentiate between active and passive forms of euthanasia.

○ Discuss the role of a hospice in managing the care of terminally-ill patients.

Overview

Many Americans have difficulty contemplating the prospect of dying; they simply avoid talking about the subject with others. As a result, most people don't prepare for their deaths by having wills and advance directives or by discussing their wishes with family members. Decisions concerning property distribution, life-prolonging procedures, organ donation, and funeral wishes need to be made as early as possible, preferably before one is terminally ill. When preparing to make decisions concerning dying and death, law professor Alex Capron asks people to focus on their values, objectives, and feelings. One question that Capron thinks people must address is "[How] do you feel about the prolongation of life itself?"

In the past, physicians were reluctant to tell terminally ill patients that they were dying. Today, physicians generally think that patients have the right to know the truth about their conditions, and they should participate in medical decision making, particularly in decisions about how to manage pain.

Patients who fear dying in pain or are in pain may ask physicians to end their lives. Many physicians, however, are uncomfortable with patients' or their families' demands for active euthanasia. According to the experts in "Final Chapter," modern technological advancements make it possible to control pain effectively so dying patients can be comfortable and coherent. Rather than seek help to end their lives, patients who have only a few months to live can enroll in hospice care programs that include pain management services. Hospice care also reduces dying patients' concerns about being abandoned or isolated during this final stage of living.

Assignments

○ Review Chapter 15, "Aging, Dying, and Death," particularly pages 433–447, in Alters & Schiff, *Essential Concepts for Healthy Living*, 4th edition. You may find it helpful to take notes on your reading. Then read the Learning Objectives and Overview for this lesson. Review the Key Terms below.

○ Scan the Video Viewing Questions, and then watch the video program for Lesson 24, "Final Chapter."

○ After watching the video, answer the Video Viewing Questions and assess your learning with the Self-Test.

○ If you haven't done so already, complete the activities for Chapter 15 in the workbook that accompanies the textbook. Your instructor may use these activities as assignments.

Key Terms

The following terms and those defined in Chapter 15 are important to your understanding of this unit.

advance directive — A document describing the extent of medical care that a person wants to have if he or she becomes incapacitated. Living wills and durable power of attorney documents are examples of advance directives.

durable power of attorney — A type of advance directive that appoints an individual who would make decisions for a person who is incapacitated.

hospice — Health care specifically designed to give emotional support and pain relief for terminally ill patients in the final stage of life.

palliative — Pertaining to treatments that relieve pain and suffering.

resuscitation — Using artificial respiration and cardiac massage to revive or sustain a dying person.

Video Viewing Questions

1. Today, terminally ill Americans often die in a hospital or a long term care facility. One hundred years ago, where did Americans usually die? For a person who is terminally ill, what are the advantages of dying at home?

2. What is the purpose of having an advance directive? What aspects of critical and terminal care need to be discussed with family members or close associates while one is still capable of making decisions? What factors need to be considered before a person chooses someone to serve as his or her durable power of attorney?

3. Dr. Mosqueda states that one of the most important things we can do as healthcare professionals is help people through the dying process. How can health care professionals help people who are going through the process of dying? Why do many physicians tell patients that they are terminally ill? How do children react to being told they are going to die?

4. What are the typical emotions that a terminally ill person experiences? According to Dr. Goldstein, what is the number one fear of dying persons? What fear is the second greatest concern of dying persons? What is palliative care?

5. What is active euthanasia? According to law professor Alex Capron, the courts recognize that it is not wrong to stop treatment that leads to a patient's death or to continue treatment that has been rejected. If physicians will not make the decision to stop treating a patient, who should? What can physicians do to reduce the likelihood that dying patients will want active euthanasia?

6. What is hospice care? What are the benefits of hospice care?

Self-Test

Multiple Choice

1. Which of the following statements is true?
   a. Most Americans prepare wills and advance directives before dying.
   b. An advance directive indicates which relatives inherit valuable items that belonged to the deceased person.
   c. By preparing advance directives, people can indicate their health care preferences in case they become unable to make these decisions.
   d. The purpose of a durable power of attorney is to identify who will manage an estate when the owner dies.

2. According to Dr. Korsch, studies of dying children indicate that they
   a. adapt better to dying if they know about their poor prognosis than if they are not given the information.
   b. ignore information concerning their medical outlooks because they can't understand it.
   c. don't care about dying.
   d. deliberately isolate themselves from parents and health care practitioners when they know they're going to die.

3. Kübler-Ross noted five emotional responses that people typically experience when they learn that they are terminally ill. Which of the following responses is not one that Kübler-Ross discussed?

a. Denial

b. Euphoria

c. Depression

d. Anger

4. According to RN Donald Bustle, the terminally ill person often experiences _____ as his or her condition deteriorates and pain increases.

a. euphoria

b. fear

c. hunger

d. serenity

5. Dr. Goldstein states that the number one fear of terminally-ill persons is

a. dying while asleep.

b. losing control over decision making.

c. having excessive medical bills.

d. being abandoned.

6. Which of the following statements is false?

a. Terminally ill people fear the pain that is often associated with dying.

b. Palliative care refers to the management of the physical and emotional pain of dying.

c. There are medical experts who specialize in pain control and management.

d. American physicians treat pain too aggressively, usually overmedicating terminally ill patients as a result.

7. According to Alex Capron, the decision to maintain life support for a dying person rests principally with

a. the administrators of the patient's hospital.

b. a board of doctors who are on staff at the patient's hospital.

c. the patient and his or her family.

d. a group of clergy from the patient's home town.

8. Terminally ill patients who have only a few months to live can receive palliative care at home or in a special facility. This type of health care is called

a. hospice care.

b. bereavement.

c. mourning.

d. intensive care.

Short Answer

9. Discuss the advantages of preparing an advance directive for health care.

10. Active euthanasia or physician-assisted suicide is a very controversial subject. Discuss measures that could reduce dying patients' demands for physician-assisted suicide.

Expanded Analysis

1. When Jerome was 45 years old, he was in good health. At that time, he decided that he did not want any "medical heroics" to extend his life should he become incapacitated. To carry out his wishes, Jerome prepared an advance directive, which he showed to and discussed with family members. After placing the advance directive in a file drawer, Jerome forgot about it. Twenty years later, he had a major heart attack. The attack weakened him, but he was determined to live life as fully as possible. When he was 77 years old, he experienced another severe heart attack and was hospitalized in the intensive care unit. The physicians who were caring for Jerome told his family that his heart was weakening and he was terminally ill. His family requested that the physicians follow Jerome's wishes by not using any extraordinary measures to extend his life. The physicians, however, told family members that Jerome gave them different instructions when he entered the unit. Jerome told his physicians to make every effort possible to keep him alive. His family members were shocked and confused by Jerome's change of instructions. Explain what Jerome and his family could have done to avoid such confusion at this time.

2. If you were very ill, would you want to be told by your physician that you had a terminal disease? Explain why you would or would not want to know.

3. Your parents are 80 years old and not in the best of health. Discuss how you would organize a family conference to determine their wishes concerning terminal care.

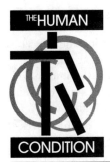

25

The Medical Marketplace

Learning Objectives

Upon completing this lesson, you should be familiar with the facts and concepts presented in the lesson and should be able to:

○ Differentiate between private and public forms of health insurance; between HMOs and PPOs.

○ Describe what information a consumer needs to obtain before selecting a health insurance plan or a primary care physician.

○ Recognize the critical role the patient plays in making health and medical decisions.

○ Outline some strategies to improve communication with health care professionals, and apply them when you next visit the doctor.

Overview

What kinds of health care do you need? Which health care practitioners should you use? And most important, how will your health care be financed? If you haven't had to consider your health insurance options by now, you probably will in the near future.

Many companies provide private health insurance as a benefit for their full-time employees. Most employers limit the number of health insurance plans from which their workers can select. Furthermore, workers often have to pay a share of their health insurance premiums as well as office visit and pharmacy co-pays.

Under the fee-for-service system, providers of health care services and supplies set their own charges. Additionally, health care practitioners decide what kinds of medical care are necessary for their patients, such as certain diagnostic tests or surgical procedures. Consumers usually like this type of payment plan because they can choose any qualified health care provider, including specialists. However, the fee-for-service method of paying for medical care is usually more expensive than other forms of payment, and there are few incentives to keep medical costs under control.

Many workers who are eligible for health insurance participate in managed care programs. The two most common types of managed care plans are health maintenance organizations (HMOs) and preferred provider organizations (PPOs). These for-profit organizations contract with various health care practitioners and facilities to provide medical care and supplies at fixed costs. Health care practitioners who participate in HMOs receive a set amount of money for each patient enrolled in the plan, regardless of the extent of their care. This form of reimbursement for medical care is called capitation.

HMOs emphasize preventive health care services such as annual checkups, Pap smears, mammograms, and vaccinations. According to Mark Laret, Director of the University of California–Irvine, Medical Center, "HMOs work well for patients who need routine services, preventive care, simple things. HMOs do not work well for patients who need advanced therapy, cancer treatments, advanced surgery and so forth."

One drawback of traditional HMOs is that patients must receive most of their care from the limited number of practitioners who work in facilities operated by the HMO. Some HMOs require participants to pay an additional amount if they want to obtain medical care from a more extensive list of participating physicians. Furthermore, physicians and patients who participate in managed care organizations usually have little control over medical decision making.

Health care practitioners and hospitals that contract with PPOs charge the insurance companies less for their services than those who are not on the list of preferred providers. If members of a PPO use practitioners or hospitals that are not participants in the plan, they may have to pay all health care costs out-of-pocket.

Public Financing of Health Care

Medicare is a public health insurance program that covers nearly all people over 65 years of age in the United States. The Social Security Administration (SSA) enrolls elderly persons in Medicare and collects payments. Medicare benefits are also available for certain disabled people who are younger than 65 years old and for individuals suffering from kidney failure.

To obtain their medical benefits, Medicare recipients may choose the fee-for-service option, or they may choose to participate in managed care programs such as HMOs. Since Medicare does not pay all medical expenses, the government encourages recipients to buy supplemental health insurance.

Medicaid is a state-operated program that provides health care benefits for qualified low-income persons, regardless of age. Pregnant women, disabled or blind persons, and aged individuals who meet state eligibility guidelines can receive such benefits. State and federal governments share the expense of providing Medicaid services. To reduce health care costs, many states require managed care options for Medicaid participants, particularly HMOs.

Building Trust

Patients need to develop and maintain a trusting relationship with their primary health care physicians. Communication between patient and physician is an important element of this relationship. Health care practitioners can facilitate the communication process by treating the patient as a whole person.

Another way physicians can build strong relationships with their patients is to involve them in the medical decision making process. Coscarelli points out that patients should have the right to make choices. But the patient is not the expert, so it is really important that physicians and patients work together."

The issue of who decides what is best for the patient—the patient or the patient's physician—has changed over the years. At one time, physicians made all the decisions. Today, physicians are more likely to act in partnership with their patients. Alex Capron, Professor of Law and Medicine at the University of Southern California, notes "…there has to be a deep participation by both parties in that process. And it's not one dominating." In some cases, patients may want to include alternative medical therapies with their conventional treatments; in others, patients may decide that no treatment is the best course of action. By communicating effectively with their patients, physicians can understand why patients make these choices and can respect their wishes.

Choosing Health Care Practitioners

Choosing suitable medical practitioners for you and your family can be difficult, especially if you are enrolled in an HMO. Most managed health care programs limit the consumer's choices; enrollees usually select physicians, dentists, and hospitals from an approved list of providers.

One way to find good health care providers is to ask family members or friends for their recommendations. Then you can check your health insurance plan's list of providers to see if the names of recommended practitioners and hospitals are included. Dr. David Goldstein, Chief of General Internal Medicine at the University of Southern California Department of Medicine, recommends academic medical centers for the best care. Physicians at these facilities usually are aware of the latest scientific and medical knowledge in their fields of practice. Your goal should be finding a primary care practitioner whom you trust and can communicate with easily.

Assignments

○ Read the Learning Objectives and Overview for this lesson. Review the Key Terms below.

○ Scan the Video Viewing Questions, and then watch the video program for Lesson 25, "Medical Marketplace."

○ After watching the video, answer the Video Viewing Questions and assess your learning with the Self-Test.

Key Terms

The following terms are important to your understanding of this unit.

HMOs	— Health Maintenance Organizations; organizations that provide managed care to patients, paying set fees to health care providers.
Medicaid	— A state-operated program that provides health care benefits to qualified low-income people, regardless of age. The federal government partially funds Medicaid.

| Medicare | — A public health insurance program that covers nearly all elderly citizens in the United States. |
| post adjuvant | — The period of time after a disease has been treated with medications that enhance the action of other drugs. |

Video Viewing Questions

1. Many health insurance programs require patients to pay part of the costs of doctor visits, diagnostic tests, and medications. What are some drawbacks of having patients share these costs?

2. When choosing a health insurance plan, what are some questions that consumers need to have answered? How does Mark Laret think health care costs will be financed in the future?

3. What factors facilitate the relationship between patients and their health care practitioners?

4. How can patients and physicians work together to achieve the best results?

5. How can traditional Chinese medical practices be integrated into Western medical practices? What are the limitations of Chinese medicine?

6. How does the medical community control the quality of care provided by its professionals?

Self-Test

Multiple Choice

1. Which of the following statements is true?
   a. Health insurance plans that include co-pays require participants to share the cost of office visits and prescription drugs.
   b. HMOs provide incentives to physicians who refer patients to specialists.
   c. The majority of Americans are dissatisfied with their physicians.
   d. Medicare participants must be at least 40 years of age.

2. The public health insurance program that covers nearly all elderly Americans is called
   a. medicaid.
   b. medihealth.
   c. medicare.
   d. mediplan.

3. The state-operated program that provides health care benefits for qualified low-income people, regardless of their age, is
   a. medicaid.
   b. medihealth.
   c. medicare.
   d. mediplan.

4. Bob participates in a managed care health insurance plan offered by his employer. Every time he goes to the doctor, Bob only has to a $10 fee. This fee is a
   a. copayment.
   b. deductible.
   c. premium.
   d. fee-for-service.

5. Eliot doesn't need to obtain referrals from a primary care physician whenever he wants to see specialists. He simply chooses physicians from the phone book, makes his appointments, and goes to see the specialists. His health insurance covers the costs of office visits and medical testing. This type of health insurance plan is called
   a. cost sharing.
   b. managed care.
   c. medicare.
   d. fee-for-service.

6. Which of the following statements is true?
   a. The fee-for-service system of paying for medical care is usually less expensive than other forms of payment.
   b. Physicians set their own charges for medical care if they charge on a fee-for-service basis.
   c. People who enroll in fee-for-service medical care payment plans have little freedom to choose their medical practitioners.
   d. Since the early 1900s, managed health care plans have been the traditional system of paying for medical care in the United States.

7. HMOs work well for patients who need certain health care services. Which of the following health care services is *not* handled well by HMOs?
   a. Routine check-ups
   b. Preventive care
   c. Annual physical examinations
   d. Advanced therapies

8. James would like to find a well-trained primary care physician who will provide him with excellent routine care. Which of the following types of physicians should he choose?
   a. Endocrinologist
   b. General internist
   c. Orthopedic surgeon
   d. Gastroenterologist

9. Physicians make errors in diagnosis. Medical experts, such as Dr. Koop, the former Surgeon General of the United States, blame such errors on
   a. poor medical training of American physicians.
   b. low quality of medical technology in the United States.
   c. lack of communication between patient and physician.
   d. use of out-of-date diagnostic equipment.

10. Which of the following medical practices is not a form of traditional Chinese medical care?
    a. Acupuncture
    b. Massage
    c. Radiation therapy
    d. Tai chi

Short Answer

11. You have been offered a full time job with a large company. The company provides health insurance coverage for its workers. Discuss the questions that you need to have answered when choosing health insurance.

12. Compare fee-for-service health insurance plans with HMOs. What are the strengths and weaknesses of each system of paying for health care?

Expanded Analysis

1. For routine and preventive types of health care, HMOs provide good coverage. Why don't HMOs work as well for medical care for advanced therapies?

2. Mr. Laret thinks that a combination of managed care and fee-for-service health insurance will be offered in the future. Do you think this is a good idea? Explain why or why not.

3. Massage, acupuncture, and tai chi are alternative medical therapies. Why do many people who are using conventional medical treatments also use alternative therapies?

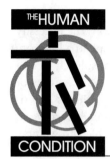

26

What Price?

Learning Objectives

Upon completing this lesson, you should be familiar with the facts and concepts presented in the lesson and should be able to:

○ Discuss the inequities in health care and other problems that exist as a result of the way health care is financed in the United States.

○ Explain why health costs are increasing in this country.

○ Account for the early "success" of managed care in comparison to the difficulties health professionals and patients are now experiencing.

○ Analyze the methods proposed for providing basic health insurance for all Americans. Select the one you believe has the greatest chance for success, and give the reasons for your choice.

Overview

Cutting-edge scientific research and technological advancements contribute to making the U.S. health care system one of the best in the world. High quality health care, however, is expensive. Some 50 years ago, health care costs comprised five percent or less of gross domestic expenditures in the United States; these costs now comprise about 15 percent of the nation's gross domestic expenditures. This rate of growth is expected to increase as consumers demand the latest diagnostic and treatment procedures for their health care. Despite the availability of quality health care, many Americans express concerns about the rising cost of care, medications, and health insurance premiums.

To finance their health care, many Americans rely heavily on private and public health insurance programs. Since health insurance plans limit coverage and do not pay for every expense, consumers must pay a share as out-of-pocket costs. A chronic illness, long-term hospitalization, or nursing home stay can rapidly deplete their financial resources. Many Americans, however, have inadequate health insurance coverage; an estimated 44 million people in the United States have no health insurance at all.

Out-of-Control Costs

As just mentioned, health care costs comprise about 15 percent of this country's gross domestic expenditures. Dr. Gerard Anderson, a professor in the School of Public Health at Johns Hopkins University, questions the necessity of spending so much money on health care. He notes, "We spend a lot more on technology than other countries...how much of that is absolutely necessary? How much of it results in a better outcome?" Alex Capron, a professor of Law and Medicine at the University of Southern California, thinks American consumers are responsible for the rising costs of health care. According to Capron, "...we take conditions that were previously untreatable and we now can treat them. Well, that's good, but what we've done is sort of increased the overall level of expectation of what healthcare can provide." He points out that healthcare practitioners often use expensive medical technologies to improve people's quality of life rather than to save lives. Americans expect this kind of care, and they expect their health insurance to pay for it.

Initially, Americans embraced managed health care as a way of reducing medical costs by cutting out frivolous, unnecessary treatments. Over time, however, many people have become disenchanted with this system of health care. Managed care has not held down the cost of medical care in the United States, and many physicians who participate in managed care programs complain that they've had to sacrifice too much of their control over diagnostic and treatment procedures. According to Dr. William Schwartz, a Professor of Medicine at the University of Southern California School of Medicine, "[Doctors are] not able to do all the things that they should do, and now the economic incentive for a managed-care doctor is very small in terms of doing more. In fact, he can be punished or penalized, or dropped from the plan, if he does too much in the eyes of the managed care program."

No Simple Solution

Although politicians, experts, and private citizens have suggested various ways to solve the health care crisis in the United States, nothing has been done. According to Alex Capron, "...every American [should have] access, equitable access, to the healthcare system, that that's a social obligation." Capron thinks that access to health care begins with employer-provided health insurance. Mark Laret, the director of the University of California–Irvine, Medical Center, thinks that the federal government eventually will provide universal health insurance. But two critical questions remain unanswered: Who will pay for universal health insurance and when will the program be adopted?

Assignments

O Read the Learning Objectives and Overview for this lesson. Review the Key Terms below.

O Scan the Video Viewing Questions, and then watch the video program for Lesson 26, "What Price?"

O After watching the video, answer the Video Viewing Questions and assess your learning with the Self-Test.

Key Terms

The following terms are important to your understanding of this unit.

Medicaid — A state-operated program that provides health care benefits for qualified low-income people of all ages. The federal government partially funds Medicaid.

Medicare — A public health insurance program that covers nearly all elderly citizens in the United States.

Video Viewing Questions

1. What factors contribute to the high cost of health care in the United States? Why are many Americans not covered by health insurance?

2. What are some of the disparities in the availability of health care in the U.S.? What are some hospitals doing to keep from losing money?

3. Gerard Anderson and Alex Capron raise questions concerning the usefulness and need for certain medical treatments. What are their concerns?

4. During the 1980s, the managed care movement swept the U.S. health care system. What is managed care, and why did it become popular? Why are many Americans now dissatisfied with managed care programs?

5. Since no health insurance program pays for every type of medical care, Americans can expect rationing of care. In the United States, how is medical care rationed? Rationing medical care poses some serious questions for health insurance providers. Is there a fair way for insurers to determine what kinds of care are more valuable than others?

6. Alex Capron and Mark Laret have different views concerning how healthcare will be financed in the future. What are their views?

Self-Test

1. Over 40 million Americans have no health insurance. Which of the following segments of the population is highly unprotected?
   a. School teachers
   b. Auto industry workers
   c. College students
   d. Young children

Multiple Choice

2. Which of the following statements is true about health care in the United States?
   a. The majority of elderly people are not covered by health insurance.
   b. Advertising by drug companies is partially to blame for the high cost of medications.
   c. Ninety percent of health care costs is spent on doctors and hospitals.
   d. Regardless of the disorder, the federal government provides financial aid for treatments.

3. During the 1970s and early 1980s, which of the following conditions contributed to the rise of managed healthcare programs in the United States?
   a. In 1983, American doctors went on strike, demanding a managed care system.
   b. The American Medical Association changed its recommendations concerning the education of doctors.
   c. Doctors were complaining that they were spending too much time with their patients.
   d. Physicians were requesting too many unnecessary diagnostic tests.

4. Which of the following statements is true concerning the U.S. health care system?
   a. The percentage of gross domestic expenditures for health care increased since the 1950s.
   b. Today, Americans pay for about 75 percent of the cost of medical care directly as out-of-pocket expenses.
   c. The use of medical technologies such as CT scans and MRIs has helped to keep medical costs down.
   d. Americans spend less on health care than people in other developed nations.

5. According to Dr. Schwartz, the original concept of managed care was to
   a. reduce the number of medical specialists.
   b. increase the emergency room caseloads of public hospitals.
   c. eliminate frivolous and unnecessary forms of medical care.
   d. decrease the size of medical malpractice awards.

6. Which of the following statements applies to the managed care system in the United States?
   a. Today's physicians have more control over diagnostic testing and treatment options than they did 30 years ago.
   b. Physicians who order too many tests can be penalized or dropped by managed healthcare insurance providers.
   c. From 1985 to the present, the managed care system has reduced health care costs by reducing waste and inefficiency.
   d. American physicians rely less on modern technologies such as MRIs than doctors in other countries.

7. Health insurance companies control their costs by rationing care. Compared to other countries, what factor largely determines who receives adequate health care in the United States?
   a. The patient's ability to pay for treatment
   b. The patient's chances of surviving as a result of the treatment
   c. The likelihood that the treatment will reduce the impact of an illness
   d. The age of the patient

8. In most countries, employers provide health insurance for their workers. This is called
   a. fee-for-insurance.
   b. social insurance.
   c. managed care insurance.
   d. co-payment insurance.

9. Explain why health care costs have increased steadily in the United States since the 1980s.

10. Discuss reasons why many Americans are dissatisfied with their managed care health insurance plans.

11. In "What Price?" Alex Capron and Mark Laret suggest two different ways that adequate health insurance can be provided for all Americans. Discuss how their universal health insurance plans would be financed.

Short Answer

Expanded Analysis

1. Healthcare systems do not pay for every service that patients want; therefore, consumers should expect some rationing of medical care. Giving health insurance companies the ability to decide whether a treatment is useful raises some serious ethical questions. In many instances, health insurers will not pay for procedures that may extend people's lives. If you had to make the decision to exclude certain procedures from being covered, which ones would you exclude? Explain why.

2. Great Britain's healthcare system is quite different from the system in the United States. What are the advantages and disadvantages of the British healthcare system? Do you think such a system would work well in the United States? Explain why or why not.

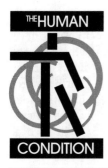

Answer Key

1 – The Fabric of Health

1. c   video
2. b   video
3. d   video
4. a   video
5. c   video
6. d   video
7. a   video
8. d   video
9. a   video
10. b   video

11. Answers will vary. Gene expression may result in negative health effects such as developing physical abnormalities and disorders, as well as certain psychological problems. On the other hand, gene expression may produce positive health effects such as longevity and a strong immune system. Behavioral and developmental factors, however, play a major role in determining whether or not and the extent to which many genes are expressed. (video)

12. Life span is the maximum number of years that a member of a species can live. Life expectancy is the average number of years that an individual born in a particular year can expect to live. When a high proportion of younger members of a population die, the life expectancy of that population drops. As more people in a population survive childhood and live to be very old, life expectancy rises. (video; p. 5)

2 – In Human Terms

1. c   video
2. a   video
3. d   video
4. b   video
5. c   video

6. a   video
7. a   video

8. Many physicians who work for Doctors Without Borders in war-torn or disease-ravaged countries are from other nations. When the medical care practitioners arrive in an area, the residents often distrust them. It takes some time before the physicians gain their clients' trust. Furthermore, these physicians often work under difficult conditions because of inadequate medical facilities and a lack of supplies. Additionally, certain cultural traditions can interfere with the medical practitioners' ability to heal patients and prevent the spread of diseases. (video)

9. Providing high quality care and adequate attention to the growing number of low-income people who seek treatment at Venice Family Clinic are among the obstacles faced by the clinic's health care workers. Although clinic workers strive to get to know their clients and meet each one's needs, such care often takes a lot of time. So clients may have to wait a long time before they can see a health care practitioner. Since the clinic is staffed by volunteers, another challenge is finding specialists, such as nephrologists, who can provide their services on a consistent basis. (video)

10. Many of the patients who seek treatment at the Venice Family Clinic do not have health insurance. So they can't afford primary care, including regular checkups. As a result, they come to the clinic when their illnesses have progressed to severe stages. Additionally, low-income people often can't afford to take good care of themselves because they're struggling to pay the rent or buy food for their children. Regardless of income, people who have unhealthy lifestyles are more likely to be severely affected by illness than people who are committed to practicing healthy life. (video)

3 – State of Mind

1. b   video
2. c   video; p. 35
3. a   video; p. 35
4. c   video; p. 40
5. b   video; p. 43
6. c   video; pp. 43–44
7. b   video
8. a   video; p. 36
9. c   video; pp. 41–42
10. d   video; p. 42
11. b   video
12. d   video

13. Dr. Leuchter says, "Obviously depressed mood is the most common manifestation of depression...[other manifestations include] loss of energy, difficulty functioning on the job, feeling like you can't cope...feeling like you just want to withdraw and do nothing." From time to time, you probably have had these feelings. How could you tell if your feelings are normal "ups and downs" or signs of depression? (video; pp. 32–33)

14. Abnormal behavior can occur when parts of the brain are damaged by injury or disease. In many instances, however, people suffer from mental illnesses because their personalities interfere with their ability to cope effectively with their environment. In other cases, genetic factors that influence brain chemistry can produce abnormal behavioral responses to situations. (video; p. 35)

15. People suffering from either anorexia nervosa or bulimia nervosa have a morbid fear of becoming fat. Additionally, individuals with eating disorders are depressed and display compulsive behavior. Medical practitioners often treat both disorders with a combination of medication, psychotherapy, and nutritional counseling. The most obvious difference between the two conditions is body weight. People with anorexia nervosa are extremely underweight, whereas people who suffer from bulimia nervosa usually have normal body weight. (video; pp. 41–42)

4 – Lives in Balance

1. c video
2. a video
3. a video
4. b video. p. 66
5. d video; p. 38
6. c video
7. c video
8. d video

9. Arthur is dealing effectively with everyday stressors if he can identify the sources of stress in his life and analyze whether he feels capable of handling the stress. Then Arthur needs to consider his stressors as problems that he can solve. If he can follow these steps whenever stressful situations arise, he has the skills to manage his stress effectively. (video; pp. 62–63)

10. Meg is able to transform the problems that she encounters into opportunities for personal growth. She probably has a strong sense of commitment and control. Furthermore, she sees stressful situations as challenging problems that she can solve. (video)

11. After such a catastrophic event, survivors usually experience a variety of emotions. Initially, survivors may cry and express a sense of denial of what has taken place. Feelings of anger tend to follow the denial. For example, survivors may express anger at God for not sparing their homes or the government for not providing aid quickly. In some instances, victims of the storm may be euphoric as they realize they survived the event. Others, however, become depressed when they see how much they have lost. Feelings of guilt are also typical. For example, victims might think that if they had heeded the earliest storm warnings, they might have had enough time to save neighbors, pets, or treasured items. Over time, however, most victims accept what has happened and are able to move on with their lives. (video)

5 – Behind Closed Doors

1. d   video
2. b   video; p. 80
3. a   video; p. 88
4. b   video
5. c   video; p. 84
6. b   video
7. a   video

8. Numerous factors are associated with the risk of juvenile violence. Children who are exposed to violence in the home are more likely to be violent. Children who live in poverty and have low self-esteem may be susceptible to joining a gang. The accessibility of guns and drugs increases the likelihood that an angry, frustrated youth will respond violently, especially when conflict arises between gangs.

    Communities and schools can establish conflict resolution programs that teach "it's not OK to use violence to solve conflicts." Additionally, communities can reduce the risk of youth violence by providing jobs and activities to keep young people busy and productive. (video; pp. 81–82)

9. Public health experts describe violence as an "epidemic" because violence is not confined to inner cities or poverty-stricken areas. Like an infectious disease that does not discriminate between a rich person and a poor person, violent behavior spreads throughout all segments of the population. (video)

10. Children who witness domestic violence are at risk of perpetuating the violence as adults. They are also at risk of abusing drugs, being arrested for criminal behavior, and abusing their own children. (video; pp. 76–77)

6 – It's Personal

1. b   video
2. b   video
3. d   video; p. 142
4. c   video
5. d   video; p. 142
6. a   video
7. b   p. 133

8. Answers may vary, but you will need to consider what information is age-appropriate for your children. Appropriate picture books about sexuality are usually available at local libraries to read and show to your children. Older children need to know more than basic biological facts about the reproductive systems. They need to learn about healthy relationships, sexual diversity, and the risks associated with sexual behavior. (video; pp. 142–154)

9. A person who is sexually ignorant may be unable to appreciate the diversity of sexual behavior. As a result, this person may be intolerant of other people's sexual behaviors and attitudes, have misunderstandings with a partner concerning sexual matters, and experience difficulties forming healthy relationships. A person who lacks knowledge about the complex nature of sexual orientation may be intolerant of homosexuals. Sexual ignorance can also increase one's risk of having unwanted pregnancies or contracting sexually transmitted infections. (video)

10. Although scientific evidence indicates that biological factors play a major role in the determination of an individual's sexual orientation, people often think homosexuality is simply a matter of personal choice. Many heterosexuals oppose homosexuality for religious reasons. As a result, the homosexual lifestyle is vilified, and homosexuals experience hatred and discrimination. So it seems unlikely that a person would choose to endure such treatment. (video; p. 142)

7 – Risky Business

1. c   video
2. b   video; p. 120
3. a   video
4. b   video
5. a   video; pp. 114–115
6. b   video; p. 409
7. c   video; p. 408
8. d   pp. 121–122
9. c   video; p. 402
10. a   video

11. When taken as directed, oral contraceptives are very effective as a method of birth control. The contraceptive effects of birth control pills do not persist after they are discontinued, which is good for couples who decide to have children. Women who use oral contraceptives have lower risks of benign breast masses and ovarian and uterine cancer. "The Pill" also reduces the likelihood of painful menstrual cramps and heavy menstrual bleeding. For women approaching menopause, oral contraceptives help regularize menstrual periods. The negative effects of taking oral contraceptives include increased risk of blood clots, psychological depression, and headaches. (video; p. 120)

12. Answers will vary but should include information about the reliability of abstinence and other methods of contraception, sexually transmitted infections, and proper use of condoms. (video; pp. 114–121 and 398–415)

8 – The Code

1. d   video
2. a   video
3. a   video

4. b video; p. 380
5. d video; p. 414
6. c video; p. 413
7. b video
8. c video
9. b video

10. According to Dr. Dean Hamer, Chief of Gene Structure and Regulation at the National Cancer Institute, genes determine about 90 to 95 percent of a person's physical characteristics. Although genes influence a person's "internal" features (for example, personality, the kind of person one is, intelligence, and sense of humor), environment modifies their contribution to these traits. (video)

11. By having information about their genetic make up, people could know which conditions they are likely to develop as they age and possibly take steps to prevent or forestall the diseases. A couple could decide whether or not to have children, especially if they have genes that code for deadly diseases that have no cures. On the other hand, a person who has such genetic information could have difficulty finding employment and obtaining health insurance, especially if this person has genes for serious illnesses that are costly to treat. If employers have access to potential workers' genetic information, they might not hire persons who carry certain genes for serious illnesses because their health insurance costs could increase. (video)

12. Prenatal screening can detect physical defects or genetic abnormalities that affect a fetus. Some conditions can be treated *in utero;* others can be treated soon after birth. In cases involving severe fetal abnormalities, parents can decide to terminate or continue the pregnancy. Parents who choose to continue the pregnancy may have time to prepare emotionally and financially for their offspring's special needs. (video)

9 – Haley or Matthew's Story

1. b video
2. c video
3. c video; p. 103
4. d video
5. c video
6. a video
7. c video
8. b video
9. c video
10. d video; p. 113
11. a video; p. 104
12. a p. 250

13. By skipping breakfast and not eating after dinner, Cindy is fasting for long periods of time. Pregnant women who fast increase their risk of having premature or low birth-weight babies. Weight gain is very important during pregnancy. Therefore, Cindy needs to consume adequate amounts of calories, eat breakfast, and avoid fasting. (video)

14. There are several reasons why this couple cannot conceive. Omar's sperm count may be too low to fertilize an egg. Catlin may not be ovulating or she may have blocked oviducts. Women over 30 years of age are less fertile than younger women. Thus, Catlin's fertility may have begun to decline naturally if she is over 30 years of age. Excess stress also contributes to infertility, especially in women. In some instances, however, physicians may be unable to explain why a couple cannot conceive. (video; p. 113)

15. Breast-feeding provides the best formula for an infant. Breast-fed babies are less likely to suffer from dehydration and diarrhea than formula-fed babies. Additionally breast-fed infants have fewer respiratory tract, ear, and digestive tract infections than formula-fed babies. Furthermore, the skin-to-skin contact that occurs when a woman breast-feeds her baby may facilitate the emotional attachment process between mother and child. (video)

10 – The Growing Years

1. c video
2. c video
3. b video
4. b video
5. a video
6. c video
7. c video
8. b video
9. c video
10. c video

11. Children are at risk of gaining weight if they are sedentary and eat too much fatty food. Many children are sedentary because their neighborhoods are crime-ridden and lack safe play areas. In these situations, concerned parents have their children play indoors and participate in sedentary activities such as watching television. Furthermore, many parents are too busy to plan or prepare low-fat, nutritious meals for their families. As a result, parents buy fast foods because they are relatively inexpensive, convenient, and appeal to children. Children are unlikely to adopt healthy lifestyles if their parents are not good role models and do not encourage good eating and physical activity habits. (video)

12. Children need to be physically active because such activity strengthens their bones and reduces their risk of obesity, type II diabetes and atherosclerosis. Furthermore, children who enjoy being physically active are likely to continue engaging in this lifestyle as they grow up. (video)

13. Reading to children provides intellectual stimulation that helps their brains develop. Picture books are especially enjoyable for children because they stimulate their imaginations. Children who are read to can learn their language as they connect words with pictures. By being read to in childhood, children may develop a lifelong love of reading. Additionally, families can spend some relaxing, enjoyable time together while engaged in reading stories. (video)

11 – Web of Addiction

1. b   video
2. d   video
3. c   video
4. d   video
5. b   video; p. 171
6. c   video; p. 170
7. a   video; p. 174
8. c   video; p. 174
9. a   video
10. c   video; p. 170
11. b   video
12. b   video; p. 181

13. Cecily may have inherited the gene for novelty seeking because she shows the signs of a thrill-seeker. Inheriting the gene for novelty seeking increases the likelihood that a person will try potentially dangerous activities. Alicia's lack of interest in potentially dangerous situations indicates that she may have the gene that is not associated with thrill-seeking. Therefore, Alicia may have a lower risk than Cecily of becoming addicted to mind-altering drugs. (video)

14. People who live in impoverished, drug-infested environments have a high risk of addiction. For these individuals, drug use is often a means of escape. Some people may use drugs because they lack information about the consequences of drug use or they believe the drugs are not harmful or addictive. Young people often have difficulty resisting offers to use drugs because of peer pressure. In addition to environmental influences, genetic factors play a role in drug addiction. Inheriting the gene for a novelty-seeking personality may predispose a person to abuse drugs because he or she gets a thrill from the behavior. Additionally, people who are clinically depressed or have other psychological illnesses are at risk of using drugs as a way of escaping their problems or feeling better. It is likely that most cases of drug addiction are the result of more than one factor influencing the susceptible person's decision-making process. (video)

15. Treatments for drug addiction include individual and group counseling, and if necessary, medications such as methadone to ease withdrawal symptoms. Counseling can help drug abusers identify what makes them crave drugs and find alternatives to drug use. Additionally, counseling can teach drug abusers how to avoid situations that foster substance abuse and find positive ways of coping with their stress and feelings of anger and frustration. (video; pp. 180–181)

12 – Feels So Good (Hurts So Bad)

1. a   video
2. c   video
3. a   video
4. d   video; p. 190

5. b   video
6. d   video
7. a   p. 204
8. c   video
9. b   video
10. a   video; p. 205
11. d   video
12. a   video

13. An alcoholic has a strong compulsion to drink alcohol and cannot control the amount and timing of his or her drinks. The alcoholic neglects other interests, because drinking and recovering from the effects of alcohol take up a considerable amount of time. Additionally, the alcoholic shows signs of tolerance and withdrawal. People who are addicted to alcohol continue to drink despite the drug's effects on their health and well being. (video; p. 191)

14. At high doses, alcohol can cause nausea and vomiting. Long-term heavy drinking can cause memory loss and impairment, vitamin deficiency, liver damage, inflammation of the pancreas, cardiovascular disease, and cancers of the esophagus, liver, and stomach. Alcohol also affects the functioning of the reproductive and immune systems. (video; pp. 196–200)

15. Cigarette smoking is the leading cause of preventable deaths in the United States. Tobacco use is responsible for about 30 percent of all cancer deaths that occur annually in this country. Additionally, tobacco use contributes to heart attack, stroke, emphysema, chronic bronchitis, osteoporosis, and gum disease. (video; pp. 209–212)

13 – What You Don't Know

1. a   video; p. 466
2. b   video
3. c   video
4. d   video
5. c   video
6. a   video; p. 464
7. c   video; p. 463
8. b   video
9. d   video; p. 466
10. a   video
11. b   video; p. 456
12. c   video

13. The villagers should boil their water before drinking it or filter it through clean, finely woven cloth. Certain chemicals can be added to water that kill the parasites but leave the water safe for people to drink. The best way of preventing this infection is to help people obtain safe underground sources of water, such as from a bore hole well. (video)

14. You should make sure the company is reputable and its employees are licensed to use pesticides. Ask the exterminator to show you his or her license. If the person is not licensed, your dwelling may not get an effective or safe treatment to eradicate the pests. Before the house is treated, have the exterminator provide a written description of the pesticide that will be used. If you have questions concerning the safe use of the pesticide, contact the EPA. Learn what you can do to minimize the risks the pesticide may pose to you and your family, especially young children. (video)

15. It is likely that the pesticide methyl parathion is present in the home's carpeting, draperies, flooring, and wallboards. Once the chemical has soaked into the housing material, there is no way to wash it out. Therefore, these materials will have to be removed and replaced. The child's toys would also be contaminated and have to be destroyed. (video)

14 – Food for Thought

1. a video; p. 226
2. b p. 226
3. b video; pp. 238–239
4. c p. 227
5. c p. 235
6. d video; p. 247
7. a p. 236
8. c video; p. 235
9. b video; p. 231
10. c video; p. 235
11. a video; p. 238
12. b p. 231

13. In this food, fat contributes 75 percent of the calories. (Multiply 15 grams of fat by nine calories per gram, which equals 135 calories from fat. Divide 135 calories from fat by 180 calories in the serving.) Thus, 75 percent of the calories are from fat. Health experts recommend that people consume no more than 30 percent of their total daily caloric intake from fat. You may not want to eat this food because it would contribute such a large percentage of your daily fat. (pp. 245–246)

14. Joe did not eat enough fruits, vegetables, and grain products. His dairy food intake is high fat and marginal. Answers will vary but should include foods that would meet the recommended number of servings of foods from those groups. (pp. 243–245)

15. To improve his diet, Joe needs to eat fewer fatty foods like doughnuts, nacho sauce, pizza, chips, and steak. He should eat more nutrient-dense foods such as fruits, vegetables, and whole grain products. Additionally, he could replace high fat dairy products with low-fat calcium rich foods such as yogurt or non-fat milk. (pp. 243–245)

15 – Weighing In

1. d   video; p. 258
2. a   video; p. 260
3. b   p. 264
4. d   video; p. 264
5. c   video; p. 270
6. a   p. 274–276
7. a   video
8. d   video; p. 270
9. a   video
10. a   video
11. c   video; p. 261
12. b   p. 258

13. The distribution of the excessive body fat influences its health risks. People who have most of their body fat distributed in the middle of their bodies (android pattern or "apple shape") are more likely to have the serious health problems associated with obesity than those who have most of their fat distributed below the waist (gynecoid pattern or "pear shape). People can determine if they have gynecoid or android patterns of fat distribution by measuring their waist and hip circumferences with a tape measure. If the waistline measurement is greater than the hip measurement, the person probably has an android pattern of fat distribution; if the waistline is less than the hip measurement, the person probably has a gynecoid pattern. (video; pp. 264–265)

14. Most people regain the lost weight because they lost the weight rapidly while following fad diets, but returned to their usual eating and exercise behaviors. Also, the body's fat mass may influence appetite. When fat cells lose some of their fat, they signal the brain to feel hungry, which makes it difficult for a formerly overweight person to control his or her food intake and maintain the lower weight. (video; pp. 269–270)

15. To help Bill analyze the diet plan, you would need to ask him several questions. For example is the plan medically sound (safe) to follow without a physician's supervision? Does it include a nutritious calorie-reduced diet plan? Is it adaptable to one's psychological, cultural, and social needs? Does the plan promote regular exercise and does the diet emphasize fruits and vegetables and low-fat foods? Does the plan provide suggestions for enlisting the support of others? Weight reduction plans that include these and other features (shown in the box on page 240 of your textbook) are likely to result in safe weight loss and long term maintenance of the lost weight. (video; pp. 269–270 and 274–276)

16 – Working It Out

1. a   p. 285
2. c   video; p. 285
3. d   video; p. 308
4. b   video
5. c   video; p. 288

6. b   p. 299
7. c   video
8. d   p. 288
9. c   video
10. b   p. 291
11. d   p. 288
12. a   p. 291

13. Exercising for longer than an hour produces no additional health benefits and can increase the risk of injury. (video)

14. Judy needs to consider her goals, what physical activities she would like to do and is capable of doing, and which activities she will engage in for a lifetime. For example, if her goals are to increase her cardiorespiratory fitness, lose 15 pounds of fat, and tone her muscles, she needs to choose aerobic, stretching, and weight lifting activities that she will practice regularly. Furthermore, she should decide when to practice her regimen and whether she needs special equipment to perform her favorite activities. (video; pp. 302–303)

15. The pros of involving Mandy in physical activities would be to help the child burn off energy, which could keep her from gaining too much body fat. Performing aerobic activities would also improve the functioning of her heart and lungs, which may reduce the likelihood that she'll develop atherosclerosis later in life. She might enjoy participating with others in a team sports activity and become very good at the sport if she continues the activity as she gets older. Such activities might develop her strength, endurance, balance, speed, and coordination. Marie and Mike, however, should be concerned about the cons of placing too much emphasis on their young child to excel in athletics or other strenuous physical activities. By rushing Mandy into a physically demanding activity before her body is mature enough to perform it safely, they might injure their daughter physically and psychologically. Furthermore, Mandy will dread participating in the activity if it is not fun and she is forced to participate. Under these circumstances, she may develop an aversion to such activities in the future. (video)

17 – Germ Warfare

1. a   video
2. d   video
3. b   video
4. a   video
5. c   video
6. a   video
7. c   video
8. c   video
9. b   video
10. a   video

11. People with viral infections should not expect their physicians to prescribe antibiotics because these medicines are not effective against viruses. When taking an antibiotic, it is important to follow the physician's

instructions and take them in the full amount over the course of treatment. This often means taking the antibiotic even after the symptoms have improved and one is feeling better. (video)

12. There are many ways to avoid infectious diseases. Several vaccines are available that prevent infectious diseases such as measles, mumps, and whooping cough. You should make sure that you and your children are immunized against those infectious diseases. Taking good care of yourself is another way to prevent infections. Moderate exercise, for example, can strengthen your immune system. By properly cooking and handling foods, you can reduce the likelihood of contracting food-borne illnesses. (video; pp. 394–395, 402)

18 – The Modern Plague

1. b   video; pp. 400–401
2. c   video
3. d   video; p. 398
4. d   video
5. b   video; p. 401
6. c   video
7. a   video
8. b   video
9. d   video

10. HIV can enter the body when blood or sexual secretions from an infected person are exchanged. This can occur when one has unprotected sexual intercourse with a person who is infected with the virus, shares IV needles that have been used by a person infected with HIV, or has a transfusion with blood from an infected person. During pregnancy, the virus can pass from an infected mother's bloodstream into her fetus's blood. The virus can also pass from mother to infant during delivery or breast-feeding. (video; p. 401)

11. When HIV entered the DNA of Arthur's immune system's T4 cells, the virus was able to remain in these cells for years. Although Arthur initially appeared to be healthy, the virus was making copies of itself within his T4 cells. Eventually, large numbers of infected T4 cells died, and Arthur's body could not make enough T4 cells to replace them. Without those cells, his immune system could no longer recognize pathogens and mount an effective immune response. He developed AIDS, a deadly disease characterized by a variety of opportunistic bacterial, fungal, and viral infections. (video; p. 400)

12. Many people think AIDS is a disease that affects only homosexual males; therefore, they may not take adequate precautions to avoid contracting HIV. Furthermore, people may think that HIV/AIDS is no longer a major public health problem in the United States, now that the death rate from AIDS has decreased. However, rates of HIV infection are increasing in this country, especially among women. (video)

19 – Heart of the Matter

1. d   video; p. 326
2. a   video; p. 319
3. c   video
4. a   video
5. b   video; p. 325
6. b   video
7. d   video; p. 326
8. c   video; p. 326
9. c   video; p. 321
10. b   p. 319
11. d   video; p. 323
12. a   video; p. 319

13. A person with a healthy level of total cholesterol can have atherosclerosis because total cholesterol does not provide information about the amounts of the different lipoproteins that carry cholesterol in the blood. LDL is the lipoprotein that carries cholesterol into tissues, including the cells that line arteries. High LDL levels contribute to plaque build-up in coronary and other arteries. Thus, one can have a total cholesterol level that is in the healthy range but still have a high risk of atherosclerosis if his or her LDL cholesterol level is too high. (video; pp. 325–326)

14. You can tell Marissa that coronary bypass surgery involves surgically removing veins from her body, usually leg veins, and grafting the veins to blocked coronary arteries. The veins carry blood around the blockages. Bypassing blocked section of the arteries allows blood to reach heart muscle that is beyond the blockage. (video; pp. 320–321)

15. Although Samantha does not have a family history of atherosclerosis, she has other characteristics and lifestyle behaviors that place her at risk for the condition. She should be concerned about her health because the negative effects of risk factors such as cigarette smoking and excess body weight accumulate, increasing her risk of heart disease. Additionally, her age is a factor; she is post-menopausal, which increases her risk. (video; pp. 325–328)

20 – Brain Attack

1. c   video
2. b   video
3. c   video; p. 328
4. d   video; p. 324
5. a   p. 324
6. a   p. 324
7. d   video
8. d   video; p. 319
9. a   video; p. 324
10. c   video; p. 327
11. b   video; p. 327

12. The physician will recommend that you learn to relax and change your diet. You could alter your diet by reducing salt and fat intake. If your blood homocysteine levels are elevated, your physician may recommend that you take vitamins B-12, B-6, and folic acid. Losing excess weight and exercising help reduce blood pressure also. (video; p. 331)

13. If you think someone is having a stroke, check for other suddenly occurring symptoms and signs such as severe headache, speech problems, and unsteady walking. According to Dr. Saver, you should call 911 or drive the man to an emergency room, if the signs and symptoms don't subside within 10 minutes. (video; p. 324)

14. There could be several reasons why Phyllis recovered faster than her grandfather. Phyllis' stroke may not have been as extensive as her grandfather's. Also the brains of younger stroke victims may be more capable of recovering from such damage than older brains. As a new mother, Phyllis may have been more motivated to recover from her stroke than her grandfather. (video)

21 – diagnosis: Cancer

1. a video; p. 344
2. d video; p. 345
3. a video; p. 347
4. b video; p. 344
5. d video; pp. 363–364
6. c video; pp. 351–356
7. e video; p. 360
8. c video; pp. 344–345
9. d video; p. 345
10. a p. 344
11. b p. 345

12. Cancer results from mutations that occur to certain genes. When mutations occur to genes that control cell growth, the cell is unable to regulate its rate of growth. When tumor-suppressor genes mutate, they are not able to stop cells from growing. In either case, cell growth takes place without the normal "brakes," and the affected cell is cancerous. (video; pp. 344–345)

13. Early detection of cancer greatly improves one's chances of survival, because the cancerous tumor can be treated before some of its cells metastasize. Once the cancer has spread to other tissues, it becomes more difficult to treat effectively. (video; pp. 364–365)

14. Information from epidemiological studies can shed light on the risks and benefits of living under certain environmental conditions or engaging in certain practices. In the United States, for example, the prevalence of nasopharyngeal cancer is higher in certain Asian populations than in white and African-American populations. By comparing information concerning the lifestyle practices and environments of each population sub-

group, significant differences may become evident. Those differences can help scientists determine risk factors and preventive measures for nasopharyngeal cancer. (video)

22 – Living with Cancer

1. b video; p. 365
2. a video
3. a video
4. d video
5. c video; p. 350
6. a video
7. b video
8. c video
9. a video; p. 365
10. d video; p. 349
11. c video; p. 350
12. d p. 350

13. Herceptin selectively interferes with the functioning of cancer cells because it binds to a specific protein that is on the cancer cell's membrane. By binding to this protein, Herceptin interferes with the cell's ability to receive signals to grow. This treatment for breast cancer is unique because it targets the specific protein that is made by the cancer cell and interferes with its functioning. The antibody does not affect the growth of cells with the normal gene. (video)

14. The results of clinical trials provide researchers with information about the effectiveness and safety of a chemotherapy. Although a treatment may be effective, it may produce serious side effects that limit its usefulness. Therefore, researchers can determine the benefits and risks of treatments by analyzing the results of clinical trials. (video)

15. Support groups provide opportunities for cancer patients to share their experiences with others who are battling the disease. Furthermore, cancer patients can learn coping strategies as well as information about side effects of treatments by interacting with support group members. (video)

23 – Age Happens

1. b video
2. a video; p. 428
3. b video
4. c video
5. d video
6. c video; p. 428
7. a video; p. 429
8. b video; pp. 430–431
9. d video; p. 430
10. a video

11. Heredity influences longevity because genes control many aspects of health as well as the changes that occur with the aging process. Genes that code for good health and longevity are passed down from generation to generation. Lifestyle factors, however, can override the potential for longevity. For example, a young man has ancestors who lived to be 100 years old, but he smokes, drinks excess alcohol, and doesn't exercise regularly. This man has a high risk of lung cancer, liver disease, and obesity. These conditions are likely to result in the man's premature death. (video; pp. 427–428)

12. When choosing exercises that are appropriate for the residents of the facility, it is important to consider the type of exercise. Appropriate physical activities or exercises should suit the person's abilities and limitations. Because older adults have slower reaction times than younger people and often have some osteoarthritis, physical activities that involve rapid or awkward movements, such as judo, are not appropriate. Another important consideration is the accessibility of exercise facilities. If the nearest swimming pool or golf course is 20 miles away, and the older adult does not have a car, swimming or playing golf are not suitable forms of exercise for this person. Finally, the instructions for the exercise should be simple enough for the aged person to remember and follow. (video)

13. You might want to ask Maria why she thinks her mother has Alzheimer's disease? For example, has Maria noticed any significant changes in her mother's ability to remember and process information during the past year? Can her mother recognize people and remember their names and relationships to her? Does she know where she is? Can she read a map or a clock? Maria needs to know that not all memory loss is due to Alzheimer's disease. Strokes are a major cause of dementia. If Maria's mother has high blood pressure, she may have had one or more small strokes. Also, it would be helpful to know if her mother is taking several medications or has had surgery recently, since polypharmacy can cause dementia. (video; pp. 430–431)

24 – Final Chapter

1. c video; p. 441
2. a video
3. b pp. 336–337
4. b video
5. d video
6. d video
7. c video
8. a video; pp. 438–439

9. By preparing an advance directive for health care, an individual indicates his or her wishes concerning terminal health care should this person become incapacitated and unable to make such decisions. Thus, family members and physicians can follow the dying person's wishes without

forcing them to wonder what kind of care he or she would have wanted. An advance directive also enables one to choose a person who will "speak" for him or her under such conditions. (video, pp. 441–442)

10. The demand for active euthanasia could be reduced if physicians treat dying patients so they can be comfortable and coherent. For example, physicians should use palliative care measures to keep the patient as pain free as possible. (video)

25 – The Medical Marketplace

1. a video
2. c video
3. a video
4. a video
5. d video
6. b video
7. d video
8. b video
9. c video
10. c video

11. There are many questions that consumers need to consider when choosing health insurance. How much is it going to cost? What are your choices? Can you choose a fee-for-service or managed care plan? If you already have a primary care physician, can you continue to use this practitioner? If you have a medical problem that requires a specialist, do you have to obtain a referral from your primary care physician before you can see the specialist? Is there a limit to the number of visits you can have with a specialist? What should you do in case of an emergency? What happens if the health insurance plan does not cover treatment that could save your life? If the health insurance administrators refuse to cover life-saving treatment, how can you appeal the decision? (video)

12. Physicians who participate in fee-for-service health insurance programs establish their own fees and charge health insurance companies accordingly. Unlike physicians who participate in managed care programs, fee-for-service physicians have more control over their services because they can order any test or treatment that they consider necessary. Under the fee-for-service system, patients have more choices of physicians, including specialists. Under the managed health care system of payment, physicians are paid a set amount per patient, regardless of how much care the patient requires. Managed care physicians may receive incentives for helping to keep down the cost of health care; they may be penalized if they order too many expensive tests or treatments. Patients enrolled in managed care programs must choose primary care physicians from a limited list of participating practitioners. Their primary care physicians decide whether or not to refer patients to specialists. Although people who participate in managed care programs find it easy to obtain routine care and medical check-ups, they do not find it as easy to seek more advanced therapies from specialists. (video)

26 – What Price?

1. d video
2. b video
3. d video
4. a video
5. c video
6. b video
7. a video
8. b video

9. Over the past 25 years, health care costs have increased in the United States primarily because American consumers expect their physicians to use the latest technological advances to diagnose and treat conditions. Many of the new tests and therapies are costly. Additionally, drug companies use expensive advertising campaigns to introduce new medications to the public. The pharmaceutical companies pass on this cost to consumers by charging high prices for prescription medications. (video)

10. Many Americans are dissatisfied with managed care because they feel that their health care choices are too limited. For example, they can't go to their doctor or see a specialist or make a trip to the emergency room whenever they want because the care may not be covered. Additionally, patients often feel that their physicians don't have enough time to spend with them. Physicians are unhappy with managed care because they no longer have control over much of the medical decision-making. What they can do for their patients is limited. There are no financial incentives for them to do more for their patients; on the contrary, they can even be penalized for doing more. (video)

11. Although many experts agree that universal health insurance is necessary, how to pay for the insurance is an issue. In most countries, it is the responsibility of employers to offer health insurance. U.S. employers would probably need incentives, such as tax breaks, to provide insurance coverage. Other ways to fund a universal health insurance program could be through a progressive income tax or through payroll deduction, in which a percentage of an employee's wages would go into a special fund for health insurance. (video)